Poisoned at the Grocery Store Copy

Why Shopping Fresh Is Not Enough to Escape a Toxic Food Supply

Marko Vovk

Paperback: ISBN 978-1-969955-16-7
Ebook: ISBN 978-1-969955-17-4

Cover Design by Marko Vovk (Draft 1 on 12/11/25 Draft 2 12-30-25))

Book Edit: Non-Human: (Autocrit, Word, Atticus, Perplexity, Grammarly Plus, Book Brush, Word Art)

Interior Design by Marko Vovk Book Cover by Marko Vovk Images by Google, Book Brush, Paint, Marko Vovk, Perplexity

Final Edit by Marko Vovk (Some minor inconsistencies may exist) Printed in USA

Disclaimer and Special Note from the Author

DISCLAIMER

This book is for informational and educational purposes only. It is not medical, legal, financial, or professional advice, and it is not a substitute for consultation with qualified healthcare or other licensed professionals. Always seek the guidance of your physician or other qualified provider with any questions you have about your health, diet, or environment, and never disregard professional advice or delay seeking it because of something you have read here. The author and publisher disclaim any liability for actions taken or not taken based on the contents of this book.

Special Note from the Author

These books are independently written and produced without a large editorial team. Many titles in this series are marked as Draft 1 or Draft 2, with the goal of releasing a fully revised Draft 3 edition in the future as new information, research, and reader feedback become available. One advantage of modern self-publishing is the ability to update and refine a book quickly.

If you notice errors, have suggestions, or believe something important should be added or clarified, you are warmly invited to email your comments so future updates can be more accurate and useful. Thoughtful, constructive feedback and fair, honest reviews are always appreciated and help guide which chapters and topics are improved next.

Much of this material is also shared free on the author's YouTube channels under "ClevelandMarko," where book text, narrated content, and AI-generated images and videos are used to reach more people.

Contents

Introduction

Food today is supposed to be safer and smarter. Yet more people feel sick, drained, and tied to pills than their parents. That question would not leave me alone. Poisoned at the Grocery Store is the result of that hunt for answers.

For years doctors and culture said disease was mostly heredity or bad luck. In my forties, a gout diagnosis turned each step into fire. Food clearly drove each flare and long night. The place that feeds families also loads bodies with chemicals never chosen.

"Shop the perimeter." The advice sounded simple as carts rolled past glass cases. I filled a cart with meat, dairy, produce, and baked goods. For a while, the symptoms eased, then the pain and swelling returned. My body reacted against items wrapped in health claims. The outer ring hid factories, additives, and toxic packaging behind glass. Shopping for produce and chilled items alone could not escape a toxic supply. I stopped behaving like a casual buyer and began to investigate.

In the cereal aisle, I read every label under cheerful mascots. Many boxes that promised whole grain lacked real fiber and were laden with sugar. Colors came from pigments, and vitamins came from labs, not soil. "At least it has vitamins." The label still stretched on with words no child could pronounce.

Cake mixes, cookies, macaroni dinners, and instant noodles told the same story. Cheap flours, industrial oils, heavy sugars, and long chains of additives filled every panel. Then came shelves of cans, packages, and frozen meals. Metal containers often used inner coatings that could leak hormone disruptors into soup and beans.

Plastic wraps, trays, and bottles could transfer residues into meat, cheese, sauces, and leftovers. Heat, storage time, and fat pulled those chemicals deeper into each bite. Frozen dinners, pizzas, and breakfast sandwiches depended on preservatives and dyes for survival. Engineered oils modified texture and shelf life long before any home oven.

Shock did not end with boxes and metal and plastic. It reached the foods once trusted most. Behind counters, I saw animals raised on grain, drugs, and cramped pens. Those bodies became products with nitrites, phosphates, fillers, and flavor boosters never mentioned in country stories.

"Is this from a local farm?" A hand waved toward the back room, then reached for the following order. At the chilled seafood displays, fillets came from enclosures packed with medicated feed. Other species carried mercury and plastic fragments from tainted water.

In the produce section, wax and residue clung to apples, peppers, and berries. Color stayed bright while travel and storage drained real vitality. Many vegetables and fruits began life in fields treated with herbicides and insecticides. Fungicides settled into skin and flesh and stayed through washing.

Seeds often were bred or altered for yield and storage life. Minerals, authentic flavor, and strength dropped down the priority list. "It looks beautiful, so it must be great." The display glowed while the story behind it stayed hidden. Labels that promised purity also demanded a closer look. Logos for organic foods could still rest on items with certain additives. Oversight weakened when profit pressure rose. Stands at open markets that claim to be local and pure, sometimes reselling wholesale produce and fake honey.

"Where is the farm?" A finger pointed toward distant hills and moved to the next customer. Pretty gardens behind the tables often served as props, not as real supplies. The deeper the search went, the clearer the pattern became. The system moves product first and guards human bodies second. No single villain controls this web of shortcuts and deals. Life for most people does not include herds, orchards, and private wells. Work, family, rent, and time limits change each choice instead.

This book does not worship perfection or demand extreme purity. It offers tools and clear sight in the world that exists now. One question drives every chapter: what can change today. Each section explores that question in a different aisle or case. Small shifts matter more than slogans. Changing even ten percent of what goes into the cart can cut pain, step by step, those choices can calm inflammation and lower risk. The same building that once pulled you toward trouble can become neutral ground.

Most items there push sugar into bread, sauces, snacks, and drinks. Wheat appears in meal after meal, often in stripped and altered forms. Preservatives, pesticides, fungicides, plastic particles, and engineered ingredients ride along. No one has tested that complete mixture together over a lifetime.

We eat it at breakfast, lunch, and dinner, then wonder why disease feels closer each year. Lessons came through pain, failed experiments, and long walks under harsh lights. Poisoned at the Grocery Store is the map that was wished for at the beginning. It points to traps, to pockets of real nourishment, and to better paths one cart at a time.

Chapter One

Franken Food Fiesta: The Boxed Food Trap

CHEMISTRY IS PURE CHEMICALS. Grocery stores pack boxes with food engineered in labs. They use bisphenol A, phthalates, styrene, formaldehyde, benzene, vinyl chloride, antimony trioxide, acrylamide, ammonia, sodium hydroxide, titanium dioxide, polyethylene, polypropylene, polystyrene, polyethylene terephthalate, epoxy resins, talc, calcium carbonate, and silicone. These chemicals hold boxes together and make them look clean. Some escape the packaging and join your meal.

Food sits in boxes and meets their walls, especially with air and time. High humidity, rising heat, and long storage invite chemicals to migrate into chips, crackers, or noodles. Your breakfast might come with a sprinkle of science alongside the sugar.

PFAS means per- and polyfluoroalkyl substances. Mention of PFAS runs throughout this work and in the book PFAS: The Forever Chemicals Poisoning Water, People and Wildlife by Marko Vovk, emphasizing how deeply these chemicals invade food and daily life. It coats box interiors where it fights grease and moisture, then leaks into food during transit and storage, especially at high temperatures or humidity. Over time, these forever chemicals build up in your blood and organs, weakening immunity, slowing growth, disturbing hormones, triggering cancer, and injuring the liver. Eat from a box, swallow a forever chemical

Aisles are packed with boxed cereal, crackers, cookies, cake mix, instant noodles, mac and cheese, frozen meals, microwave popcorn, protein bars, frozen fries, pizza, pancake mix, candy, granola, boxed rice, boxed soup, brownies, baking powder, tea bags, and instant potatoes. Every box hides food that saw the lab before entering your kitchen. Grocery stores display chemistry sets dressed as dinner.

Now you walk into the cereal aisle. Mascots wave at you, colors flash, and Tony the Tiger smiles from a sweet cardboard box. The ingredient list stretches: whole grain oats, corn, rice, sugar, corn starch, brown sugar syrup, salt, tripotassium phosphate, caramel color, annatto extract, natural flavor, canola oil, sunflower oil, vitamin E, calcium carbonate, iron, zinc, niacinamide, vitamin C, calcium pantothenate, vitamin B6, riboflavin, thiamin mononitrate, folic acid, vitamin B12, vitamin A palmitate, vitamin D3. You pour a bowl and add pasteurized milk.

Every ingredient gets processed in factories. Grains are stripped of fiber, then genetically modified. Sugar spikes your blood then leaves you tired. Corn starch and oil are changed for texture.

Tripotassium phosphate supports shelf life but may harm bones and kidneys. Caramel color and annatto are not found on farms. Natural flavor means chemistry, not fruit. Vitamin E arrives through science, not almond trees. All the vitamins and minerals come from labs, not nature.

Pasteurized milk endures high heat that destroys enzymes and alters proteins. Milk may contain antibiotics and hormones from factory farms. Calcium and protein survive, but much is lost. Milk fat can speed up aging, and milk sugar challenges digestion for many people. Animal studies show D-galactose in milk brings on stress and early aging.

Living only on cereal and milk becomes a struggle. Fortification may prevent some basic deficiencies. Protein scratches the surface for body repair. Healthy fats, fiber, and natural nutrients are missing. Gut bacteria fade, immunity falls, fatigue and muscle loss appear, sadness rises, and recovery slows. Within a year, serious deficiencies, infections, and weak bones can take over, especially if you begin unhealthy.

This food comes from industry, not nature. Color and vitamins are synthetic. Flavor comes from machines, not seasons. Eat only cereal and milk, and health gently slips away beneath bright colors and grinning mascots. If you count on boxes, you eat food's clever impersonator. Oreos and boxed cookies follow the pattern. Wheat flour leads every package. Sugar runs second. Palm oil, cocoa, corn syrup, leavening agents, soy lecithin, artificial flavor, salt, preservatives, and coloring fill the list. These are ingredients your ancestors never saw in the wild.

The wheat flour is stripped, bleached, and refined. It spikes blood sugar, feeds belly fat, disrupts digestion, and links to diabetes and heart disease. Little nutrition remains compared to whole grain. Sugar floods each boxed cookie. Cane sugar, corn syrup, glucose syrup, extra fructose. Sugar races through your system and knocks insulin off course, raising risks for obesity, diabetes, liver trouble, and weak teeth. Over time, sugar drains your strength and encourages sickness.

Palm oil, artificial flavors, emulsifiers, and preservatives lock in shelf life and slick texture. Palm oil jams up arteries, while emulsifiers and preservatives disturb digestion and make bad bacteria thrive. Every extra additive means greater risk and less nutrition. So when you reach for cookies in a box, look at the label. Expect flour, sugar, oil, flavor, and plenty of chemicals built for convenience, not health.

Open cake mix and you find more of the same. The lineup: enriched bleached flour, sugar, palm oil, corn syrup, baking soda, sodium aluminum phosphate, monocalcium phosphate, propylene glycol esters, modified corn starch, artificial color, artificial flavor, cellulose gum, xanthan gum, dicalcium phosphate, sodium stearoyl lactylate, and preservatives. Not one comes directly from a field or farm.

Flour here is processed, bleached, and weakened, increasing inflammation and blood sugar. Expect more fatigue, weight gain, diabetes, and heart risk. Gut health struggles as real fiber disappears.

Heavy sugar-cane, corn syrup, dextrose, high fructose corn syrup floods each mix. Sugar trips up metabolism, exhausts insulin, and stockpiles body fat. The liver suffers, dental strength drops, and risk of chronic diseases climbs.

Palm and soybean oils and chemical leaveners boost shelf life. Palm oil clogs arteries, while chemical agents irritate digestion. Emulsifiers and gums confuse gut bacteria, raising cravings. Preservatives help food last but lower immune defenses and fuel allergies or stomach issues.

Artificial colors, flavors, and stabilizers finish the story. They come from labs and petroleum, not vanilla beans or berries. Fake vanilla might even trace to the paper industry. Every slice delivers flour, sugar, chemicals, and oils. They trick the palate, but rob the body of health. Your own baking gives food. The box delivers empty promises.

Boxed mac and cheese matches the lineup. Macaroni is refined wheat flour, stripped and lifeless. This base raises blood sugar, drives inflammation, slows insulin response, and may set up diabetes or chronic fatigue. Gut health and weight stability fade.

Cheese powder is factory-made: whey, milk fat, salt, sodium phosphate, calcium phosphate, artificial color, preservatives, and flavorings. Sodium phosphate keeps things smooth, but burdens kidneys and the heart. Yellow dyes only mimic cheese. If trans fats sneak in, heart disease risk increases.

Packaging introduces phthalates and other hidden toxins. They move into the powder or pasta over time. Phthalates disrupt hormones, lower fertility, and may trigger developmental issues in kids. Exposure means more risk for some, especially after frequent use. These chemicals are invisible on labels but found in the meal.

What do boxed mac and cheese deliver? Rapid carbs, sodium overload, heavy oils, colorants, and a cocktail of unwanted chemicals. It fills quickly, but it cannot heal or strengthen the body. Every forkful pumps up inflammation and disease risk. Real food gives life; the box is nutrition in disguise.

Instant noodles mimic this with speed and salt. White flour, palm oil, flavored powder, preservatives, and coloring pack each box. The noodles are soft and bland, but the health effects strike hard. Rapid carbs and easy calories raise glucose, weight, and metabolic risks. Oils drive up fat, and salt spikes up blood pressure or triggers headaches.

Flavor enhancers like MSG amplify taste but bring headaches or mood changes for many. Packaging can offer trace metals after weeks on the shelf. Most instant noodles deliver not comfort, but a recipe for chronic strain, especially when consumed often.

Pancake mix starts with bleached flour and sugar, then adds palm oil, baking powder, sodium aluminum phosphate, and artificial flavor. These ingredients spike blood sugar, promote weight gain, and strain the liver. Preservatives and emulsifiers upset digestion and damage healthy gut bacteria, while artificial colors and flavors come from labs, not fields.

Boxed pancakes and noodles combine inflammation, poor insulin response, blood vessel wear, and unwanted pounds. Additives tip allergy and hormone balance, while comfort gives way to slow sickness or unpredictable symptoms.

Stroll down the center aisles and see the banquet of boxed food. Mac and cheese, cake mix, crackers, cookies, and cereal line the shelves. Each box holds pancake mix, soup, pudding, noodles, waffles, bread crumbs, stuffing mix, bars, and mashed potatoes. You also pass boxed rice, brownies, muffins, sweet clusters, and popcorn.

Each package brings manufactured ingredients that promise comfort but deliver risk. Sugar, stripped flour, oil, preservatives, color, and flavoring rule what you eat

Boxes dominate the aisle. Lists stretch long, grandmothers would squint at every item. Flour moves through milling, bleaching, and chemical tanks, losing life and fiber. Sugar sneaks into snacks or "healthy" options. Oil hides in unexpected places. Flavor claims start with honey or vanilla, often ending with syrup or artificial fruit. Honey itself can be sugar mixed with pollen, passing for the real deal. Real honey is rare, expensive, and boxed brands use cheap tricks that do little for health.

Every boxed food in the store is food. It looks good, smells good, and feels right at first glance. The brain believes the trick, but the body senses emptiness. Life slips away through artificial colors, sugars, and chemical flavors. Energy drops, mood changes, illness creeps in, and inflammation surges. Eat from boxes every meal and the body cries out for nature.

Boxed foods fill far more than center aisles. They crowd freezer racks, snack displays, and the edges of every grocery store. The lesson remains: if it comes in a box and claims to nourish, snack, or treat, look closer. Factories build inventions, not food.

Chapter Two

Canned Carnage: The Poison Parade in Every Pantry

CANNED FOOD FILLS EVERY shelf from soup to vegetables and even the odd fruit cocktail. Brands like Campbell's, Bush's, Del Monte, Dinty Moore, Progresso, and store varieties like Market Pantry and Walmart's Great Value offer the same promise: "freshness" and convenience on demand. But every can's story starts in a sprawling industrial plant, not a kitchen. Before any food arrives, intense acid and caustic washes, often sodium hydroxide and phosphoric acid, scour the metal.

Every can needs a shield to stop corrosion and keep the food from spoiling. Epoxy linings with bisphenol A, bisphenol S, phthalates, and sometimes vinyl chloride or polyester are slathered inside, even for "BPA-free" brands. Tests show many cans, including major names and even some organics, still use BPA or close cousins, because regulators don't require disclosure if a substitute is used. When food is heated or sits on the shelf, these chemicals seep into soup, beans, fruit, and meats, especially when tomatoes or anything acidic is inside. Independent studies link BPA and its replacements to hormonal chaos, infertility, breast and prostate cancer, obesity, developmental delays, and ADHD.

Next comes the can-filling gauntlet. Foods are cleaned with chlorinated water, ammonia, and often glycol for "extended shelf life", the food equivalent of embalming. Water and brine can carry microplastics or traces of factory lubricants, especially if a plant runs 24/7. Fatty foods, like canned fish or potted meat, draw these chemicals in even faster. Re-heat a can or leave it in the sun, and many toxins double their presence by the time you eat.

No label says "packed in a plastic parade." Hormone disruptors slip into circulation, acting like estrogen or testosterone, confusing every cell they touch. Babies, kids, and anyone with metabolic health problems face the sharpest edge, but every bite brings risk. Even brands touting "eco" or "BPA-free" may use BPS or phthalates, often with equally bad effects. Some providers, like Amy's, Annie's, Eden Foods, and Sprouts, were noted to have safer practices, but most cans tested from grocery giants still used toxic linings in at least some of their products.

The soup aisle sparkles as the king of comfort food. Campbell's Chicken Noodle, Vegetable Beef, and Tomato Soup remain top sellers, alongside Progresso's Creamy Chicken or Chunky Steak & Potato lines. The list on a typical can: beef stock, chicken broth, water, pasta, carrots, potatoes, tomato paste, celery, sugar, salt, yeast extract, hydrolyzed soy protein, caramel color, flavoring, spices, and color. Beef or chicken stock is sourced from concentrated animal feeding operations (CAFOs); bones and scraps are boiled in massive tanks, often bringing along traces of antibiotics, pesticides, and GMO animal feeds.

Tomatoes are greenhouse types grown for bulk, not nutrition. They are blanched, peeled, cooked, and packed with citric acid, often industrially produced, not fresh juice. Salt is dumped for taste, with many soups having 700 to 900 mg per serving, about half a day's safe limit. Some Progresso and Campbell's soups exceed 1,100 mg per can. Sugar isn't just for baked beans; some "hearty" or "homestyle" flavors hide 7, 10, even 15 grams per can, which is more than a glazed doughnut.

MSG and yeast extract come next. Factory fermentation breaks down proteins or spent yeast, concentrating compounds that hype up flavor but can trigger headaches, hyperactivity, nausea, dizziness, or even allergic reactions, especially in children and those sensitive to glutamates. Soybean oil, sometimes canola or corn oil, is chemically extracted under high pressure and heat, raising its omega-6 fat and oxidation risk, prime drivers of modern inflammation.

Beans promise simplicity, but every can has a catch. Bush's, Goya, Eden, and store-label beans list water, beans, salt, sugar, calcium chloride, sometimes ethylenediaminetetraacetic acid (EDTA), and firming acids. Acid and firming agents keep kidney beans and chickpeas "bright" and intact. Sugar is common, Bush's Baked Beans or Van Camp's add 10 to 16 grams per serving, more than some cookies. Flavoring in "Boston" or "Grillin'" beans means sauces with chemicals, pork or beef "smoke," and caramel color. Calcium chloride, made with limestone and hydrochloric acid, keeps beans firm but does nothing for your health if eaten in excess.

Liver health is a silent victim, with sodium content commonly above 400 mg per serving in most brands. Tropes like "natural flavor" or "spice extract" cloak dozens of manufactured chemicals, esters, aldehydes, and solvents, designed for shelf life, not nutrition. Eden Foods is a rare major brand that commits to BPA-free, phthalate-free cans. Still, every other label in the aisle can, by law, hide the plasticizers under vague ingredient lists.

Canned fruit fools the eye and tongue. Dole, Del Monte, and generic cans start with syrup that is often more than 50% refined sugar solution. Pears, peaches, fruit cocktail, and pineapple come to you pre-boiled and packed with ascorbic and citric acid. Sugar and acid mask flavor loss from the high-heat process. Calcium chloride locks firmness but does nothing for nutrition, and excess sodium builds up after even one serving.

Color and artificial flavors are common in fruit cocktails and cherry mixes. FD&C Red 3 and Yellow 5 add fake color, both linked to allergic reactions and (in Red 3's case) animal studies indicating cancer risk. None of these colorants are needed for fruit, but help keep dull factory produce looking appealing for years.

Canned meat and fish brands, Hormel, Spam, Great Value, Starkist, Chicken of the Sea, Valley Chef, Dinty Moore, offer everything from potted meat, corned beef hash, and sardines to clams and salmon. Meats are ground, emulsified, and cooked off the bone. They are stabilized and colored with sodium nitrite and nitrate, which can form cancer-promoting nitrosamines when mixed with protein and heat. Heavy salt, smoke flavor, hydrolyzed protein, and sugar define Spam, Vienna sausages, and Dinty Moore stews.

Cans of tuna, salmon, and sardines from Chicken of the Sea or Bumble Bee include sea creatures and their own load of mercury and plastics. Most olive oil blends are heated and refined, stripping antioxidants but keeping the calories. Polyphosphates in seafood (common in store brands and imported canned shellfish) preserve a wet, bouncy texture but are linked to kidney and bone risk. Mechanically separated chicken or pork is standard in bargain pates and gravies; processed with phosphates, the result is more paste than natural muscle.

Gravy and sauces, Campbell's, Heinz, McCormick, Chef-Mate, and more, are built from beef or chicken fat, mystery stock, flour, oils, artificial mushroom powder, caramel colors, and stabilizers. Sodium phosphate is added to keep sauces pouring or spreading smoothly, with levels per serving often between 400 and 800 mg.

Open the oddball cans and the magic gets weirder. Hearts of palm from Roland, Del Monte, or Reese are picked in forests, soaked in brine or citric acid, then sent around the world. Lotus root, jackfruit, and lychees from Chaokoh and Dole take a similar journey, harvested, blanched, then sealed in syrup and preservatives. Some brands, like La Choy, add calcium propionate and benzoate preservatives to their canned Asian vegetables

Canned puddings, pie fillings, and fruit gels (Lucky Leaf, Libby's, Great Value) are mostly sugar, corn syrup, sorbitol, gums, and vanillin. Sorbitol comes from corn, is chemically treated, and can trigger cramps or diarrhea in sensitive eaters. Vanillin, the "vanilla" in canned desserts, is produced using wood pulp and other petrochemicals, not vanilla beans. Carrageenan, another common thickener in canned creams, is derived from red seaweed and has been linked to gut inflammation and possible tissue irritation.

Canned spinach, beets, and artichokes may look healthy, but store versions (Del Monte, Goya, Reese) rest in salty, acidic baths with sodium often 400 mg per serving or more. Canned olives from Lindsay and Pearls are soaked in lye or ferrous gluconate for color and texture, then stabilized with citric acid. Some canned tomatoes (Hunt's, Muir Glen) use calcium chloride and citric acid for color, risking extra calcium and acid in the diet but little extra nutrition.

Even "BPA-free" cans can be lined with polystyrene, vinyl, or polyester coatings, all of which have unclear health effects but early links to hormone and immune disruption. Studies repeatedly show raised chemical biomarkers, BPA, BPS, phthalates, tin, plastics molecules, in the urine and blood of those who regularly eat canned foods, with children showing especially high hormone disruption and asthma. Additives like titanium dioxide (sometimes in pudding and canned beans) are banned in Europe for DNA and immune risk but still appear in some U.S. brands.

If your pantry is built on cans, from Chef Boyardee ravioli to Bush's beans and Campbell's soup, you are serving yourself a side of the chemistry set. Every can delivers something extra, hidden along the way. Real food should not need this much engineering; in canned carnage, the parade of poison marches on, brand after brand, bite after bite.

Chapter Three

Plastic Wrap Roulette: Eating Food in a Toxic Tomb

PLASTIC FOOD PACKAGING IS everywhere. Boxes and cans may line the shelves, but nearly everything else sits inside clear, bendy plastic. Sandwich meat, deli cheese, nuts, berries, pasta, snacks, dips, and leftovers all hide under some form of plastic wrap, tub, pouch, or tray. Walk through any grocery store or kitchen and the chemical parade is impossible to escape.

The manufacturing starts with raw polymer pellets churned out from petrochemicals. These pellets are melted, stretched, or pressed into giant sheets or tubes. A heated mold pushes the plastic into its final shape. Common types are polyethylene, polypropylene, polystyrene, PET (polyethylene terephthalate), and PVC (polyvinyl chloride). Trays and tubs are thermoformed: sheet plastic is warmed like pizza dough, then pressed into molds. Bottles, jars, and squeezable pouches are blasted into shape in seconds, cooled, then trimmed. Before filling, the plastic is tested for leaks or cracks and often gets an extra step no one sees.

Plastic is soft, so many containers need a chemical shield to resist grease, acid, or air. Most food plastics are coated or mixed with phthalates (for flexibility), bisphenols (for strength), per- and polyfluoroalkyl substances (PFAS, for grease resistance), vinyl chloride, styrene, and sometimes PVDC or acrylic resins. These substances either sit on the container's inside walls or run through its entire structure. Colorants, UV blockers, and even antibacterial chemicals like triclosan may be added during manufacturing for "protection" or branding.

Every one of these chemicals can become a sneaky ingredient in your lunch. Plastics are not a perfect seal; they shed tiny amounts of themselves into the food that touches them. Heat is the fastest trigger: microwave a leftover or pour hot soup into a plastic tub and the molecules loosen, leaking chemicals faster. Sunlight and UV rays break chemical bonds and weaken plastic in days, not months. Ever left a water bottle in a hot car? You might taste the plastic, but what you don't taste are hormone disruptors and plasticizers dissolving into your drink.

Cold has its own tricks. Freezing makes plastics contract and get brittle, causing cracks and tiny breaks. When food expands as it freezes, pressure pulls more plasticizer out. Each thaw and refreeze moves more chemicals into your meal. Even time is an enemy: months or years of storage let plastic and its invisible friends migrate slowly into your food's oil, water, or acid.

Bisphenol A (BPA) and bisphenol S (BPS) are chemicals that can act like hormones in the body and have been linked to infertility, certain cancers, diabetes, obesity, heart disease, and developmental problems in children. Phthalates interfere with metabolism and sabotage the body's hormone signals, raising risks for obesity, ADHD, asthma, and reproductive issues. PFAS (yes, the same forever chemicals found in nonstick pans and firefighting foam) are nearly indestructible and build up in blood, liver, and kidneys, causing immune dysfunction and higher cancer rates. Vinyl chloride and styrene are both classified as human carcinogens; their presence in packaging increases the threat with every snack, meal, or sip stored in plastic.

Plastic always comes with an extra ingredient list. Researchers counting substances in common food plastics found over 900 separate chemicals, with more than forty known or probable carcinogens, many never listed on any label.

Plastics may contain antimony trioxide (used to make polyethylene terephthalate, or PET), dithiocarbamates, parabens, synthetic colorants such as Azo dyes or titanium dioxide, organophosphates, hindered phenols, and metal stabilizers, all designed to extend shelf life. Many of these substances can leach into food more easily when plastics are exposed to light, heat, or certain foods, such as tomato sauce, mayonnaise, or oil-rich dips.

If your food spent time in a plastic wrapper, it probably picked up some phthalates, bisphenols, or PFAS. These plastic-related chemicals move into food from wraps, coatings, and can linings. Clear clamshells for berries, produce bags, and sliced cheese trays can transmit bisphenols, PFAS, or styrene-based plasticizers, especially if they are left in the sun, microwaved, or reused. This exposure adds up across every meal and snack, not just what you eat once.

Inside your body, these chemicals do not just pass through. They may scramble hormone signals, block nutrients, burden the liver and kidneys, and fuel chronic inflammation. Conditions linked to plastic chemicals include thyroid disease, testicular and ovarian dysfunction, blood cancers, autoimmunity, lowered fertility, and behavioral changes in children.

Brand-names and generics alike use nearly identical materials, because cost and convenience matter more than purity. Researchers checking Walmart, Target, Dollar General, and convenience store brands found plastics just as toxic as those in fast food wrappers and big-box "eco" containers. “BPA-free” means made without bisphenol A, but claims like “BPA-free,” “microwave-safe,” and “non-toxic” usually mean one chemical was swapped for another less-studied, not necessarily less dangerous, option.

In the end, plastic food packaging is not just a container. It is a delivery system for a silent soup of science experiments and industrial leftovers. Each layer or additive is chosen to resist spoilage or cracking, but it resists health and wellness in the process. When you serve food from plastic, cold, hot, or straight off the shelf, remember that the real chemistry in your life might not be just flavor and seasoning, but the box, tub, wrap, or bottle itself.

Plastic-wrapped deli meats, hot dogs, and bacon, Oscar Mayer, Hillshire Farm, and Ball Park. are preserved with nitrites, nitrates, sodium benzoate, and citric acid. The plastic is soft and loaded with phthalates and bisphenols for flexibility and strength. Over time, these chemicals migrate into the meat, especially when exposed to heat, sunlight, or cold. Fat and salt pull even more chemical residue from the plastic, so each lunch slice brings a side of hormone disruptors and cancer risks. Eating these products regularly links to inflammation, heart disease, colorectal cancer, and hormonal imbalances.

Cheeses are often mass-produced in factories, with Sargento, Kraft, and Velveeta leading the market. Shredded, sliced, and block cheeses are packaged in polyethylene, polyvinyl chloride (PVC), or low-density polyethylene (LDPE) films, all of which can leach bisphenols, phthalates, and times vinyl chloride into the food. Cheese is processed with salt, artificial color, citric acid, and enzymes, then stabilized with anti-caking agents like cellulose or potato starch. Because cheese is high in fat, it absorbs more chemicals; benzophenone, di(2-ethylhexyl) adipate (DEHA), and other toxins more easily migrate from the plastic during storage or shipping. Over time, these chemicals can build up in the body, disrupting hormone balance, increasing cancer risk, and contributing to weight gain and digestive distress.

Condiments like ketchup, mayonnaise, mustard, and salad dressings in plastic bottles from brands such as Heinz, Hellmann's, French's, and Wish-Bone often contain sugar, salt, modified starch, citric or phosphoric acid, artificial flavors, and stabilizers. These bottles are usually made from polyethylene terephthalate (PET), high-density polyethylene (HDPE), or squeezable low-density polyethylene (LDPE), along with added colorants and UV blockers for longer shelf life.

When these bottles get hot, very cold, or sit for months, the plastic can shed chemicals such as PFAS, bisphenols, and phthalates into the sauces. Over time, these substances may disrupt gut health, harm immune cells, and contribute to diabetes, obesity, and reproductive issues, turning even a small squeeze of dressing or hot sauce into another source of unwanted chemical exposure.

Each of these supermarket staples appears "fresh" and safe. In reality, the food is being preserved and seasoned with chemicals the body treats as invaders. With every slice, squeeze, or pour, plastic packaging plays lead villain, leaching hormone disruptors and carcinogens and layering harm beneath every meal. More details on meat and plastic-wrapped protein will follow in future chapters, but every plastic-packaged food adds to the slow parade of invisible poison, with cheese and condiments right beside the deli counter.

Plastic-packaged foods crowd the center of every grocery store and line the outer edges. Sliced meats, cheeses, dips, yogurts, snacks, and condiments dominate coolers and shelves, sitting beside bread and milk in clear wraps, bags, tubs, and bottles. These products look safe and modern but are striking proof that shelf life now beats real nutrition.

Some processed foods, like packaged muffins, cheese singles, deli meats, Twinkies, and snack cakes wrapped in plastic, are so loaded with preservatives and stabilizers that they barely rot, even if left out for weeks. Shoppers sometimes joke that even mice refuse to eat them, and nature has quite literally lost interest. If animals and bugs pass it by, there is no hiding from the fact: packaged chemical food is not food.

The real magic happens inside the plastic itself. Every piece is made with blends of PET (polyethylene terephthalate), LDPE (low-density polyethylene), PVC (polyvinyl chloride), and sometimes multi-layer films that resist grease or light. Plastic containers get pumped with phthalates, bisphenols, PFAS, antimony trioxide, benzophenone, and dyes like titanium dioxide or Red 40 for color stability. UV blockers like benzophenone keep salad dressing looking sunny in a refrigerated bottle. Leaching starts slow but speeds up with heat, light, and time. When containers crack, microwave, freeze, or sweat, they deliver an invisible cocktail into your meal.

Thin plastic films on cheese use DEHA and phthalates for flexibility, these migrate especially fast into fatty slices and shreds. Meats and dips come in trays lined with anti-fog chemicals and antimicrobial agents such as triclosan or silver nanoparticles. Some "fresh" deli meats are vacuum-sealed in multilayer film loaded with stabilizers, peel-off adhesives, and oxygen scavengers. Sliced bread often sits in polyethylene bags that contain slip agents like erucamide for easy opening and softer texture. Ultra-pasteurized milk is stored in high-density polyethylene (HDPE) jugs loaded with pigments and UV blockers.

Beyond the basics, rows of hummus, guacamole, snack cheeses, granola bars, muffins, cookies, nut mixes, and dried fruit live in some of the most advanced plastics available. Vegetable snacks, carrot chips, celery sticks, grape tomatoes, are often shrink-wrapped in films coated with antifungal chemicals that can slow spoilage until the produce starts to resemble a science project. Even vegan milk and plant-based yogurt are plastic prisoners, usually nestled in polypropylene cups and PET bottles, sealed with colored lids and protected by stretch-wrap. Many of these containers were simply never designed for long-term health.

Each item brings its own set of risks. High-fructose corn syrup in ketchup, barbecue sauce, and sweet dressings gives bacteria lots to feed on; the plastic makes sure they never get a bite. Potato chips and crackers come in multi-layered pouches with aluminum, PET, and plasticizers, designed to resist air and water, not to nourish. Sliced bread and hamburger buns live in bags treated with calcium propionate and sorbate to resist mold; in some brands, a loaf will outlast anything in the produce aisle. Pre-sliced vegetables, even pre-washed salads, often carry extra preservatives, like sodium benzoate or potassium sorbate, to fight off mold and stretch the sell-by date. Several brands now use plastic infused with silver or copper ions, hoping to kill germs on contact, but the effect on human cells is still poorly understood.

Look closer, and you can find energy bars wrapped in plastics containing parabens and dithiocarbamates, snack cakes sealed in packaging loaded with antioxidants like BHT (butylated hydroxytoluene) to avoid rancidity. Some microwaveable rice and noodle meals use polyester trays sprayed with acrylic polymers and anti-fog agents, keeping sauce from drying out.

When nuts, grains, or other pantry foods develop a strange, "off" smell that many people casually call **rancid**, it is often a warning sign, not something normal to ignore. In many cases, that odor can come from a mix of rancid oils and microscopic insect contamination, including insect droppings, eggs, or fragments that build up during storage.

This can happen more easily in warm, humid conditions or when foods sit for months in unsealed bags, bins, or bulk containers. If you notice a musty, stale, or slightly sour smell, see tiny webbing, fine dust, or small insects, it is safest to throw the product away rather than eat it.

Breads, tortillas, and pita are sometimes stored in bags with propylene glycol and glycerin, both are humectants that are more at home in a chemistry lab than a bakery.

Food that doesn't rot, or food that even a mouse or a bug will not eat, is not really food. When packaging wins the war against decay, health and nutrition lose. More on veggie milk, meat, and baked goods will follow as we unmask plastic packaging's hold on our food, our bodies, and our grocery store choices.

Chapter Four

Iced Deceit: The Chilling Truth About Frozen Grocery Food

OUR MIND IS FOOLED by the word "frozen." Most of us think it means long-term storage or preserving nature's best. Sometimes that is true, but the real reason so many foods are frozen is because otherwise nobody would buy them. Brands freeze off-grade broccoli florets, broken berries, or overripe mangoes that would rot on a store shelf. Fish that never got sold at the fresh counter or meat too tough for the grill gets flash-frozen for "family value" meals, and tossed by the ton into bags bearing farm-fresh scenery.

Frozen food starts out with promises of peak ripeness and perfect texture, but it picks up more than vitamins on the way. "Mystery oils" sneak into breaded chicken, fries, breakfast sandwiches, and waffles. These oils are blends of processed soybean, canola, or palm oils, often partially hydrogenated and full of industrial trans fats, mono- and diglycerides, and synthetic antioxidants like tertiary butylhydroquinone (TBHQ) or butylated hydroxyanisole (BHA). None of these are natural or good for you; they slow spoilage for months but clog arteries, disrupt hormones, and may increase cancer risk. Even pan-cooked "crispy" finishes in the frozen aisle can be a result of deep-frying in these chemical oils before your food gets frozen and bagged.

Convenient plastics in the freezer bring along all the phthalates, bisphenols, and polymer break-down products you read about before, now made worse by the damage from freezing, thawing, and microwaving. Each step in the frozen food journey adds its own dusting of chemicals, because keeping food "fresh" in a frozen wasteland takes more than cold air.

So, beneath the icy packaging, you find food engineered for a shelf-life marathon, not for nutrition or flavor. The biggest risk in the frozen section isn't frostbite, it's what's sneaking in while your defenses and the food's are frozen solid. Frozen pizza, dinners, breakfast foods, vegetables, fruit, and ice cream all start with the promise of fast, easy meals. These frozen favorites have something else in common besides ice: they come loaded with chemical preservatives, colors, oils, and additives that do anything but nourish. Most are stripped of real nutrition during processing and freezing, then rebuilt with lab inventions and a shelf life far longer than anything natural.

The preservative roster reads like a chemistry quiz: butylated hydroxyanisole (BHA), butylated hydroxytoluene (BHT), tertiary butylhydroquinone (TBHQ), sodium benzoate, calcium propionate, sodium nitrate, and propyl gallate. Each is made from synthetic petrochemicals, not from anything found in nature. They stop mold and slow down decay, but are linked to higher cancer risk, hormone disruption, gut irritation, and sometimes even liver or kidney problems.

Many older dyes like Red 3 and Yellow 5 were removed because they cause tumors and allergy attacks. New rules in 2025 now let food companies use a wave of new super dyes, some already banned in parts of Europe. Look for names like Blue 2, Red 40, Yellow 6, and Green 3 in candies, frozen desserts, and rainbow breakfast waffles. Health groups warn parents to avoid these for kids because of cancer concerns and links to hyperactivity.

These products often include artificial flavors, high-fructose corn syrup, hydrogenated and interesterified soybean or canola oil, mono- and diglycerides, and gums like guar or xanthan. These make everything hold together, fake "freshness," and bulk up on texture and sweetness. Mystery "crispy" or "buttery" flavors are never natural fats but are blends of lab-made molecules that have been linked to headaches, metabolic syndrome, and inflammation.

Frozen fruits and vegetables, though sounding healthy, often retain synthetic pesticides from field to freezer. Common pesticides found on or in frozen produce include glyphosate, chlorpyrifos, imidacloprid, and pyrethroids, residues that survive cold, shipping, and months on the shelf. Once processed and thawed, these foods can absorb more plasticizer or color from their packaging. Each bag, box, tray, and pint from the freezer aisle is one more reminder: freezing may pause the clock, but it does not pause the chemical parade, the color wheel, or the health risks hiding in each bite

Stouffer's Lasagna with Meat & Sauce and DiGiorno Three Meat Rising Crust Pizza are icons of the frozen aisle, offering quick comfort but hiding a storm of unhealthy ingredients. These popular products are packed with sodium, processed meats, artificial colors, and preservatives like BHA and TBHQ. Their meats come cured with sodium nitrite and their sauces often include synthetic flavor boosters, while crusts and pasta bulk up on processed carbs and even trans fats.

It's not just the nutrition panel that's worrying. These meals contain dyes and colorants, Red 40, Yellow 6, Blue 2, that in earlier years caused enough cancer and hyperactivity concerns to get banned elsewhere, only to be swapped for similar dyes as food laws shifted. Modern administration changes and global food politics mean ingredient lists can morph at any time. Companies reformulate for different regions, responding to health rules, ingredients prices, or local "taste" preferences. A pizza sold in the US might have one set of additives and dyes, while its European version contains others, some safer, some just different.

Brands update recipes to dodge health scandals, meet new regulations, cut costs, or keep up with trends. Thanks to this ingredient shuffle, your favorite frozen lasagna or pizza may look the same on the outside but can be loaded with new chemicals, colors, or preservatives, sometimes more, sometimes less, but rarely good. To make sense of these shifting risks, the next section will dig into how food companies choose and change ingredients for different countries and why "what's inside" matters more than ever

Frozen dinners like pizzas, lasagnas, and chicken meals often look the same on both sides of the Atlantic, but their recipe can change dramatically depending on where you buy them. Take DiGiorno Three Meat Rising Crust Pizza, for example. In the USA, it often contains artificial colors like Red 40, Yellow 6, and Blue 2, as well as preservatives such as BHA, BHT, TBHQ, and sodium nitrite. These ingredients are allowed in America, but many are banned in Europe due to health concerns: European versions usually replace the artificial colors with plant extracts or annatto, remove sodium nitrite, and avoid preservatives linked to cancer and hormone disruption. American pizzas may even use brominated vegetable oil and titanium dioxide (used for whitening), both banned or heavily restricted in European countries for cancer and DNA risk.

This difference is not just about taste, it's about what the law allows, what health organizations recommend, and what manufacturers can get away with. Companies modify ingredient lists for every region, not only due to local regulations, but also because certain chemicals cost less, last longer, or meet popular demand for color and convenience. While Americans might get a longer shelf life, Europeans get fewer artificial preservatives and dyes, yet often pay more at the register.

As you read this book, remember: what's in your frozen dinner today can change tomorrow. Manufacturers swap out ingredients for cost, health scandals, politics, or simply because a new law passes in your town or country. The same brand may sell a healthier pizza in one place, but load it with chemicals elsewhere. Without strict rules or daring transparency, companies can put new or banned substances into your food without you learning the difference, right up until the next package lands in your cart. The only sure thing in frozen food isn't the recipe, it's the risk that comes with every scoop, slice, or bite.

Walk down the frozen grocery aisle and you get more than pizzas, dinners, and vegetables. Entire sections are frozen not for nutrition, but because companies need to keep odd, fragile, or heavily processed products sellable for months. Frozen orange juice is a prime example: popular brands like Tropicana and Minute Maid do not just squeeze oranges and freeze them. They store juice in giant tanks, strip out oxygen, and later add "flavor packs" engineered from orange peels and chemical essences to recreate the scent and taste lost in processing. These flavor packs are custom mixes, sometimes including ethyl butyrate and other lab-made chemicals, never mentioned on the ingredient label. The result is juice that tastes the same every day of the year but has lost its freshness, and picked up new chemical baggage.

Many store brands and novelties are not even true ice cream, but "frozen dairy dessert" filled with corn syrup, palm oil, mono- and diglycerides, carrageenan, artificial vanillin, and sometimes titanium dioxide for a whiter appearance. The FDA lets brands like Breyer's and store labels avoid real cream, bulking up instead with stabilizers, gums, and engineered flavors. "Vanilla" often comes from wood pulp; chocolate can arrive as cocoa with extra alkali or fake aroma chemicals. What looks and tastes like a treat may deliver hydrogenated fat, synthetic sweetness, and a dose of hidden preservatives that upset the gut, raise inflammation, and add to cancer risk.

Popsicles and frozen treats are a chemistry experiment on a stick. They start with water and sugar, then pack in artificial fruit flavors (like ethyl maltol and isoamyl acetate), intense colors (Blue 1, Red 40, Yellow 6), and gums for texture. Old dyes like Red 3 have been banned, but troubling new ones have taken their place, some linked to hyperactivity, allergies, and even tumors in animal studies. The only way these "fruit flavored" treats last for months is a cocktail of preservatives and color-fast chemicals.

Add to this a list of foods people forget: frozen burritos bulking with modified cornstarch, hydrogenated soybean oil, and TBHQ; breakfast sandwiches with engineered egg products, cheap cheese slices, and sausage loaded with sodium nitrite; frozen breaded fish fillets packed with more filler than fish; frozen potato products par-fried in seed oil baths before packaging. Even things like frozen bagels, bread, and sweet rolls use calcium propionate or potassium sorbate to resist mold in the deep freeze.

The results are not surprising. When flavor, texture, and color come from a chemical lab, nutrition is not just secondary, it's absent. Most frozen foods are not designed to nourish; they are built to last, trick the senses, and keep you coming back for convenience. As you read this, remember: food companies routinely change ingredients, colors, and additives for legal, economic, or marketing reasons, often without notice. In the next section, we will break down how international rules and shifting trends let manufacturers put new, or even untested, chemicals into frozen food, and why the safest item in the freezer might still come with an unwanted chemical surprise.

Frozen grocery food is a triumph of convenience and science, but not of real nutrition. Most of what you find in frozen meals, snacks, desserts, breakfasts, and even juice is far from the whole foods people imagine. Instead, it's engineered, loaded with preservatives like butylated hydroxyanisole, butylated hydroxytoluene, tertiary butylhydroquinone, sodium benzoate, and propyl gallate; blended with artificial flavors, gums, stabilizers, colorants, and sweeteners. Dinners and pizza can be built from low-grade meat, processed starch, mystery oils, and sauces more synthetic than real. Classic breakfasts, waffles, sandwiches, even pancakes, swap out eggs and butter for hydrogenated oil and corn syrup, while ice cream and popsicles feature corn syrup, mono- and diglycerides, vanillin from wood pulp, and industrial dyes. Even "healthy" frozen fruits and vegetables are blanched, sprayed, and shrink-wrapped, losing vitamins and picking up pesticide and microplastic residues in the process.

If you tried eating only foods from the frozen section, the results would be bleak. High consumption of ultra-processed frozen foods is linked to higher rates of obesity, diabetes, cancer, heart disease, and even cognitive decline. Preservatives and additives in these foods can disrupt gut bacteria, while high sodium, sugar, and saturated fat put strain on blood pressure, the liver, and the heart. After a year, frequent frozen meal eaters face weight gain, hypertension, poor digestion, mood swings, and decreased energy. Most of these meals lack fiber, antioxidants, and the essential nutrients needed for real health and longevity. The deeper frozen food replaces fresh in your regular diet, the more chronic illness, inflammation, and premature aging become threats close to home.

Frozen fruits and vegetables, though sounding healthy, often retain synthetic pesticides from field to freezer. Common residues include glyphosate, chlorpyrifos, imidacloprid, and pyrethroids, which survive cold, shipping, and months on the shelf. Once processed and thawed, these foods can absorb more plasticizer or color from their packaging. Each bag, box, tray, and pint in the freezer aisle is one more reminder: freezing may pause the clock, but it does not pause the chemical parade or the health risks hiding in each bite.

Chapter Five

Behind the Meat Counter: Factories, Fillers, and Health Risks

FACTORY-FARMED MEATS LIKE BEEF, pork, and lamb fill the perimeter aisles of nearly every grocery store. These animals are fed a constant diet of genetically modified corn and soy, crops engineered for fast growth and sprayed with herbicides like glyphosate. These chemicals build up in the feed and, ultimately, in the meat itself. The goal? Bigger, fatter animals in less time. GMO grains change animals' digestion, impacting their fat profile, and each step in the industrial process is designed for speed, not nutrition. Feed in most feedlots is routinely supplemented with growth-promoting additives: synthetic hormones are implanted to speed weight gain and boost marbling, and antibiotics are added, not just to fight infection, but also to make the animals grow even faster.

Let's break it down by animal. Beef cattle in conventional feedlots receive hormone implants at various stages, especially in the final months before slaughter. These hormones boost weight and muscle but also leave measurable traces in meat. Though these traces are described as "minuscule" by industry, many researchers raise concerns about hormone-sensitive cancers and reproductive disorders, especially with years of eating lots of red meat. Pork is fed GMO corn and soy daily, sometimes with a side of ractopamine, a chemical banned in 160 countries but still used in the U.S. to accelerate pork growth. Lamb, often thought of as "pure," is frequently grain-finished and can be given antibiotics in crowded pens to control disease outbreaks. This strategy isn't about health, it's about efficiency, and the result is cheaper protein that might carry a major health price.

Animals raised on fast-growing GMO grains gain more fat, but their fat is not as healthy: it is lower in omega-3s, higher in inflammatory omega-6, and heavier in saturated fat than meat from grass-fed, pasture-raised animals. Conventional beef and pork offer less vitamin E and fewer carotenoids, having lost many natural antioxidants and bioactive nutrients in the factory farm process. Worse, the acidic gut bacteria fostered by grain-fed cattle encourage more dangerous strains of E. coli, which can survive even poorly cooked burgers and quietly make people sick. For the average consumer, that means mass-market meats are more inflammatory, less heart-healthy, and add risk for diabetes, cancer, and other chronic diseases driven by inflammation.

It's not just the muscle cuts you need to worry about. Modern factory farming and processing use every part of the animal: organs, bones, skin, and fat are ground up and rendered into "Franken foods." These byproducts become the base for hot dogs, sausages, lunchmeat, meatballs, and a wide variety of processed meats, often labeled as "byproducts," "meat meal," or "bone meal" on the ingredient list. Collagen from skin and bones is boiled into gelatin for candies and desserts. Once nutrient-rich, organ meats are now diluted with starch, gums, and preservatives, making them a shadow of their natural, whole-food selves.

Even the "grass-fed" label isn't a simple guarantee of health. Not all grass-fed beef or lamb is truly pasture-raised; some animals start on grass then get shipped to feedlots for grain finishing, or graze on fields contaminated by years of pesticide use. "Grass-finished" meats are better, they offer more omega-3s, less saturated fat, and more antioxidants, but they still miss key fiber and come from the top of the food chain, where environmental toxins gather. Research shows that grass-fed cattle may even produce more methane per animal, while some "grass-fed" labeling is pure marketing, especially at bigger grocery chains.

The perimeter meat section isn't the nutrition haven it once seemed. What's for sale is more than protein, it's a mix of industrial science, growth promoters, antibiotics, and sometimes questionable animal welfare. Diets heavy in processed and factory-farmed meats lead to higher inflammation, weight gain, digestive trouble, and more risk for heart disease and cancer. Many shoppers think eating from the perimeter is "healthy," but in truth, the safety and quality of grocery store meat now depend as much on industry profits and chemistry as on farming.

Modern meat production is a maze of industrial tricks that go far beyond raising animals on pasture. Most beef, pork, and lamb in the store comes from concentrated animal feeding operations (CAFOs), where thousands of animals live crowded together, eating a steady diet of genetically modified feed and chemical additives. These feeds, engineered for speed and weight gain, are laced with antibiotics, not just to prevent disease in tight spaces, but to boost growth as well. Growth hormones, beta-agonists, and enzyme treatments banned in much of the world, are still routine in U.S. beef and pork, making animals reach market size at record speed.

The tricks don't stop once the animal is slaughtered. Processors treat muscle cuts and trimmings with a variety of chemicals. Red meat and poultry are routinely washed with chlorine, peracetic acid, or lactic acid in a bid to kill bacteria, but these chemical washes can leave residues that disrupt gut health. Meat is preserved and "enhanced" with injected salts, phosphates, sugars, colorants, and even "meat glue" enzymes (like transglutaminase), binding together scraps to form uniform steaks or roast shapes. These additives keep meat moist, artificially pink, and seemingly "fresh" for weeks, but reduce nutrition and transparency.

To maximize profit, every edible bit of the animal is used. Bones and connective tissue end up in broths, bouillon, and fillers; organs, fat, and "trimmings" become ground, emulsified, and sold as hot dogs, sausages, nuggets, and deli meats. Some byproducts are hydrolyzed into protein powders or pet food, masking both the source and quality from shoppers. If the label says "byproduct," "meat meal," or "mechanically separated," be wary, these are the leftovers of modern meat-packing. Even packaging hides secrets. High-oxygen or carbon monoxide packs keep meat red and attractive beyond its real freshness, disguising spoilage. "Enhanced" or "pre-seasoned" cuts are injected with brine and flavors to pump up weight (and sodium), often at the expense of actual nutritional value.

All of these factory practices turn the meat section into an invisible health risk. Residues from antibiotics, hormones, and chemical washes build up in our bodies and can promote antibiotic resistance, hormone disruption, gut changes, and long-term inflammation. Processed and cured meats pose an even greater danger: nitrites and chemical preservatives react with proteins to create nitrosamines, powerful carcinogens tied directly to digestive cancers and chronic disease. Every shortcut drops nutritional value, real protein is replaced by fillers, salt, fat, and mystery additives.

In short, the perimeter meat section is a far cry from purity. Modern business turns what could be wholesome food into a chemistry lab experiment. The more shortcuts, enhancers, and byproducts end up on our plates, the further we drift from real nutrition, and the more risk we take with our health. Even cuts that look "fresh" conceal a story written by boardrooms, not open pasture.

The process is even grimmer for broiler chickens. From the moment they hatch, these birds face confinement and chemical management. Born in massive hatcheries, most never see their mothers, just industrial lights and endless crowds. Tens of thousands are crammed together in sheds, unable to walk or support their bodies as they outpace normal growth. Many develop twisted legs, collapsed breast muscles, or deformed wings. Living conditions are strictly engineered for temperature and light but make no allowance for comfort or animal welfare. For chicken, profit and speed come first, health and nature last.

Chickens eat concentrated mixes of GMO corn and soy, rendered animal byproducts, and relentless feed additives, all engineered to drive maximum weight gain. Their water is medicated throughout their short lives. Antibiotics are delivered as a matter of course, not just for disease but to make them grow faster in crowded barns. Chickens are injected with vaccines (and sometimes the same types used for cattle and pigs), trying to stave off viral or bacterial outbreaks that sweep through these giant complexes.

Chemicals aren't just in their feed or water. Many chickens receive hormones (banned in some countries, legal or "overlooked" in others). Often, even after slaughter, the birds are injected with saline, dextrose, or soy oil to plump up the meat and increase weight at the checkout. In a shocking twist, some chickens headed for discount brands are processed at sea on floating factories and out of reach of EPA or FDA oversight.

Once processed, chicken is flash-frozen or doused with preservatives, then shipped to meat counters or freezer aisles across the country.

But it's not just drumsticks or breasts you're buying. Factory-farmed chicken is fully commoditized: bones and skin are ground for nuggets, patties, or hot dogs; organs are blitzed into "chicken paste" for deli meats or pet food; collagen tissues become broth cubes and "extenders." The supermarket overflows with cheap, heavily processed chicken made from every scrap and a laundry list of fillers, stabilizers, and artificial flavors.

Eating this ultra-engineered chicken leads to real health risks. Residual antibiotics and hormones disrupt digestive health, promote antibiotic resistance, and can trigger hormonal changes, especially risky for children. Processed chicken is higher in saturated fat, lower in omega-3s, and often contains less protein ounce for ounce than birds raised with natural diets. Industrially produced chicken amplifies allergies, inflammation, and metabolic problems, while early life exposure is linked to bigger risks for behavioral, developmental, and immune disorders.

In the end, that "fresh" chicken in the grocer's case is no mere cut of protein, it's the final product of genetic selection, chemical cocktails, industrial shortcuts, and regulatory loopholes. The meat is stripped of depth and nutrition, pumped up with water and additives, and finished off with health risks that come from reshaping nature for higher profit. Choosing from the meat section's location does not protect you. In the world of modern food, even wings can't fly, and quick growth always brings slow, invisible costs.

Chapter Six

Poisoned Catch: The Truth About Grocery Store Seafood

THE PERIMETER FISH COUNTER may seem like the last oasis of freshness, but that shimmering display is often anything but. More than half of all seafood eaten worldwide is now farmed, not wild-caught, and for staples like shrimp and tilapia the share climbs toward 90%. Most of it comes from Asia, especially China, Vietnam, Thailand, and Indonesia, with a growing share also raised in massive indoor tanks, ponds, or sea cages in the U.S. and Europe. Wild-caught means the seafood actually lived free in a river, lake, or ocean, caught directly from its natural habitat, but that's becoming rarer and often reserved for premium species or short supply.

Farmed fish like salmon, tilapia, catfish, shrimp, and sometimes even clams, are confined by the thousands to ponds or sea pens, eating a diet of GMO soy, corn, animal byproducts, and offal a mix not even pigs would see in nature. On top of that comes a steady diet of drugs and additives, including lab-engineered hormone-like compounds, antibiotics, and chemical antifungals to keep the teeming aquatic crowd alive. The feed itself can contain dyes, flavor agents, and various "plumping" additives to make the flesh look pink and build yield quickly for sale.

The result? Fish that can grow dramatically faster, but carry residues of everything in their feed and water. When you eat them, you're getting cancer-linked hormones, antibiotic traces, pesticide residues, metals, and chemicals with every bite, contributing to the spread of antibiotic resistance, the rise of hormone interruptions in children, and inflammatory risks tied to heart, brain, and immune problems.

Shellfish are natural "cleaners" but in the modern world, their filter-feeding exposes them to every toxin or pathogen in the water. The Chesapeake is infamous for agricultural runoff, sewage sludge, and storm overflows; parts of the Gulf of Mexico, Louisiana, and Mississippi, regularly test positive for dangerous bacteria and industrial chemicals.

Bacteria, viruses, pesticides, PFAS from firefighting foam, and microplastics all build up in mussels and oysters. In the worst cases, entire harvests have sickened thousands at a time: hepatitis from California clams, norovirus and bacterial outbreaks traced to Gulf oysters, and China's vast 1988 clam disaster when toxic dump runoff poisoned nearly 300,000 people.

Crab, crawfish, and shrimp often come from "soup" ponds nowhere near clean.

These crustaceans are frequently dyed with artificial colors and packed with sodium bisulfite, formaldehyde, or other hidden preservatives. In 2025 alone, 240 shipments of foreign shellfish and shrimp were seized by the FDA for illegal additives including formaldehyde and banned antibiotics. Astonishingly, 'wild-caught' may only mean the animals spent their last days in the wild after growing up in industrial ponds and crossing oceans to get here."

Predatory fish accumulate not only mercury, PCBs, dioxins, and arsenic, but also radioactive fallout. The radioactive bluefin tuna caught off the West Coast in 2014 had spent years migrating from Fukushima's disaster zone in Japan, yet still showed up on American tables. Shockingly, most fish sold in the U.S. isn't tested for radiation at all. The EPA and FDA only run spot checks, and there are virtually no comprehensive post-processing screens unless a major incident is suspected.

Plastics outnumber plankton in some ocean regions now. Microplastics have been detected in nearly every kind of seafood, fish, clams, oysters, even in deep sea crabs. Fish eat plastics thinking they're food, which means humans swallow plastics loaded with PCBs, pesticides, dioxins, heavy metals, and plasticizers. They are persistent and only get more toxic as they concentrate up the food chain, with scientists warning that if it's in the water, it's in the fish, and then it's in you.

Global seafood distribution is an epic shell game, where mislabeling, swaps, and fraud are common. DNA barcoding shows that up to 30% of supermarket fish is not what the label claims, often lower-quality species or farmed substitutes. There's no reliable tracking system in the U.S.; barcodes can be dodged or faked, and "fresh" fish might have been frozen in Asia a year ago, then defrosted and labeled "previously frozen" or "re-caught." By the time you choose it at the counter, its true origin and history are a murky mystery.

Processing multiplies the risks. Fish is often sent abroad for processing in countries where food safety enforcement is missing or corrupt. Fillets and shellfish are soaked in chlorine, peracetic acid, and phosphate solutions (banned in many countries) to kill bacteria, improve texture, and bulk up weight. Many crustaceans are par-boiled in chemicals before freezing and, sometimes, injected with colorants or formaldehyde. These chemicals leave residue that damages our gut flora, disrupts hormones, and in sensitive people may trigger allergies or cancer risks. Even scraps get ground up into mystery "fish sticks," broths, and fake crab; you're not just eating a fillet, but an industrial byproduct stew.

The problems extend beyond hidden poisons. Processed frozen fish in the grocery aisle can be a Frankenstein's monster: battered nuggets, fake crab, and breaded 'fish portions' bulked with starches, flavor enhancers, colorants, and spreads of ground unknown species. Ingredient lists can hide everything from soy fillers to phosphate binders, gums, and fossil-fuel-based preservatives.

Seafood's parade of foodborne crises is ongoing. Hundreds of Americans get hit each year with scombroid poisoning, massive histamine overdoses from improperly handled or unrefrigerated tuna and mackerel, with symptoms imitating a heart attack. Outbreaks of Salmonella, Listeria, and norovirus from oysters, clams, and crab are regular news, and chronic, low-grade contamination by mercury, pesticides, and PCBs are far worse, contributing silently to long-term health decay. The EPA advises children and pregnant women to avoid lake fish, limit tuna, swordfish, and king mackerel, and moderate all seafood intake because these risks barely register on package labels.

Ocean damage worsens alongside the seafood on our plates. Between 75 and 199 million tons of plastics pour into the seas annually. There are now more than 500 coastal dead zones, with 100,000+ animals dying every year from ghost nets, plastics, or chemical debris. Wild fish ingest this. Farmed fish swim in it. And what's left is a shrinking, increasingly artificial catch from a dying ecosystem.

Even the purported health benefits of seafood are eroding. Farmed fish don't get their distinctive omega-3s, those heart-healthy fats, because their feed is plant-based, not marine-based. The real mineral profile is warped: minerals are replaced by metals, and the "protein" is now watered down with saline, chemical gels, and flavor agents designed to trick your senses instead of nourish your cells.

What was once the cleanest protein on earth has been transformed into a chemistry experiment; the barcode will rarely reveal the truth, and the flavor is too often synthetic shadow play. The risks are invisible but real: hormone signals in kids gone haywire, antibiotic resistance, cancer-causing chemicals, metabolic trouble, silent allergies, and, more than anything, a world in which even the healthiest, oldest foods have become modern mysteries.

Chapter Seven

Waxed, Washed, and Worse: Grocery Fruit Exposed

FRUIT MIGHT LOOK NATURAL, but most of it is now bigger, flashier, and grown for yield. Farmers use lots of chemicals to make fruit grow fast and last longer. Apples, strawberries, grapes, and oranges get sprayed with pesticides like imidacloprid, fludioxonil, or azoxystrobin. These protect against bugs and mold but can linger even after washing.

Many store fruits get a bath or a scrub before you see them. Some, like oranges, limes, and apples, are coated with edible wax made from carnauba or petroleum. Others are washed in alkaline solutions or chemical detergents. Some fruits are dyed or painted to enhance their color: Citrus Red 2 on some orange rinds, artificial reds on Red Delicious apples, and bright dyes on maraschino cherries. If a fruit is extremely shiny, it may be sprayed or "beautified" for shelf appeal.

To keep fruit fresh for shipping and months of storage, farms use preservatives and shelf-life sprays. These can include chemical fungicides or coatings that use propylene glycol. Olives and pickles are soaked in brine with citric acid or calcium chloride to preserve color and texture. This keeps fruit looking good after long travel. Some fruit is irradiated at packing plants. Radiation helps kill bacteria and pests and delays ripening. This means your pineapple, strawberries, or apples can travel farther and last longer. Irradiation doesn't destroy nutrition or make food radioactive, but it may reduce some vitamins and change flavor for sensitive eaters. Examples include apples and papaya shipped from Hawaii or Florida.

GMOs play a huge role in modern fruit. GMO apples resist browning; GMO papayas survive ring spot virus. Pink pineapples, GMO squash, and potatoes are modified for shelf life, texture, or resistance. Genetic changes are made in labs with DNA techniques, and the traits carry through every bite. GMO fruit can, for some, trigger allergies or change the way your immune system reacts.

Critics worry about long-term effects, and some countries ban certain GMO fruits. The science is debated, but labels do not always tell the whole story. In short, today's fruit has become a science project. It is washed, sprayed, painted, and sometimes irradiated to survive travel and fit the grocery shelf. When you grab a shiny apple, you might get wax, dye, fungicides, or DNA surprises. Fruit today can impress the eye but might surprise your body, too.

The most chemically treated fruits in today's stores include strawberries, spinach, grapes, apples, cherries, nectarines, pears, peaches, and berries. These are often sprayed with multiple pesticides and fungicides to keep their color and stop spoilage. Strawberries can show over thirty pesticide residues after washing. Grapes and apples usually have wax coatings or shine-enhancing sprays added at the packing house.

The "Dirty Dozen" list from the Environmental Working Group highlights these same usual suspects, confirming how heavily treated they are and how often they also receive wax, dye, or even irradiation on top of spray residues. Fruit today has lost a lot of the nutrition it once had. Farming methods focus on yield, shelf life, and perfect appearance. From 1960 to now, apples are estimated to contain around 38% fewer key nutrients. Other fruits like oranges, strawberries, peaches, and bananas show similar losses. Minerals such as calcium, iron, and magnesium, and vitamins A and C, are much lower, sometimes even cut in half.

Over-farming stretches soil thin. Farms use the same fields every year, add chemical fertilizers, and rely on fast-growing fruit varieties. This process is good for making more fruit but bad for minerals and vitamins. Quick-growing fruit cannot pull nutrients from the earth like older varieties did. Apples in the past were sometimes eaten by worms, but that was a good sign. If worms wanted your apple, it meant there were fewer chemical sprays or coatings. Today, apples are heavily treated with pesticides and fungicides, and sometimes covered with edible wax or washed in chemical solutions. Yes, they are worm-free, but they often come coated in chemicals instead.

The color and shelf shine of fruit are now "engineered." Apples, oranges, lemons, and cherries can be painted or dyed to cover up natural blemishes and age spots. Whiter or more colorful fruit may hide chemical baths or preservation treatments. Chemicals like imidacloprid, fludioxonil, Citrus Red 2, or waxes like carnauba and polyethylene are commonly used.

In short, you might need several apples today to match the nutrition found in a single apple from the 1960s. Over-farming, chemical use, and focus on appearances have changed fruit from a true health food into a manufactured product. Next time you see a perfect apple, think twice; sometimes good fruit is ugly, and ugly fruit is better for you.

Fruit is handled by lots of people at every step. Each handoff can add germs, risking contamination and illness. In 2023, peaches, nectarines, and plums caused a deadly Listeria outbreak in the United States. Eleven people across seven states got sick, one person died, and one pregnant woman had preterm labor. Listeria can survive on fruit skin after packing and handling.

The same year, frozen organic strawberries from Baja California, Mexico, spread hepatitis A to people in several U.S. states. People ate the fruit straight or blended it in smoothies. Everyone interviewed told the CDC they ate those strawberries right before getting symptoms. Similar hepatitis A outbreaks hit from California strawberries in the 1990s. In recent cases, cantaloupe and fruit mixes with melon cubes spread Salmonella in at least fifteen states. Arizona had seven cases, and several states reported four or more. Markets involved included Aldi, where pre-cut fruit sat in open containers. Sometimes ill food handlers pack fruit, as happened in several outbreaks linked to melon, date, and orange packing plants.

In 2011, contaminated apples with Listeria sickened buyers in several states. Caramel apples became risky after Listeria survived in wax coating or got embedded during packing. Any fruit touched many times and not washed well before eating can spread bacteria or viruses. Even perfect-looking fruit can carry invisible microbes that cause major outbreaks.

Fruit used to be picked and eaten right from the branch. Today, farms grow for mass appeal and storage. Apples, strawberries, and grapes are grown for size and shine, with very little focus on true nutrition. Modern fields use chemical fertilizer, heavy irrigation, and fast-growing hybrids to push yield. The soil loses minerals and trace nutrients every year, leaving fruit looking perfect but offering less nourishment in each bite.

Chemical sprays are almost always part of the story. Apples, grapes, pears, and berries are some of the most heavily treated and often show multiple synthetic residues even after washing. After picking, fruit may also be treated with wax. Apples, citrus, and some plums get coatings of carnauba or petroleum wax to lock in color and stay glossy. Some fruits get dyes, like Citrus Red 2 on oranges and artificial red on cherries or apples. These treatments make the fruit sell better but do nothing for your health.

Storage and shipping add new risks. Fruit travels for weeks before hitting store shelves, so it is sprayed with preservatives, gassed with ethylene, or sometimes irradiated to stop mold and pests. Apples are often held in cold warehouses for months. During that time, chemicals like diphenylamine can migrate to the fruit surface or combine with wax coatings. Imported papayas and mangoes are often irradiated at the packing plant. Radiation prevents rot and pests but may lower some vitamin content and alter flavor.

Fruit can become contaminated by more than farm chemicals. Irrigation water can contain bacteria from animals or sewage. Unwashed hands, dirty bins, and packing equipment can transfer germs. Mexican strawberries and melons from multiple suppliers have triggered Salmonella outbreaks.

Heavy metals like lead and cadmium sometimes show up in fruit or in processed juices. Soil pollution and cheap packaging are to blame. Some fruit may also pick up residues from animal-based fertilizers or polluted compost. In recent years, tests have found toxic metals in popular juices made from strawberries, apples, and pineapple. In the end, perfect-looking fruit is often a sign of industrial care, not nutrition. Ugly, blemished fruit attracts worms and bugs, which often means it is safe for you to eat. Modern, mass-market fruit is more likely to be coated, colored, and gassed to look ideal.

Bad or rejected fruit rarely goes to waste. It gets sent to the pie filling and canned fruit departments, where it is covered, sweetened, and even colored. Stores use fruit with bruises, strange shapes, or dull color that supermarkets reject. After washing and slicing, these cherries, peaches, and apples are transformed into fillings for pies, puddings, jams, and fruit gels.

Canned cherries, especially maraschino cherries, give the brightest and most artificial warning signs. These are packed with sugar, corn syrup, vanillin, and thickened with gums. Red dyes such as Red 3 and Red 40 are often used for the cherry's color; they can carry benzidine, a known cancer risk. Some brands use erythrosine as a dye, which can cause phototoxicity. Preservatives like sodium benzoate and citric acid are added to keep the cherries firm and sweet as long as possible. Bisphenol A (BPA) can leach into these cherries from the can lining, affecting hormones in your body. These ingredients and chemicals may cause problems for digestion, liver function, and even cancer risk over time.

Now for a lighter warning, the mighty fruit sticker. Stickers are slapped on apples, pears, bananas, and most other fruit for store codes and branding. Sometimes, stickers are not removed and get eaten by mistake. The FDA says fruit stickers are made from non-toxic glues and plastic films. Accidentally eating one is not supposed to hurt you, but stickers are not food. If you ignore the sticker, it could sneak into a smoothie or a fruit salad and remain undigested. The sticker will pass through your body like a confused barcode. If fruit had real labels for everything in and on them, most people would prefer the sticker over all the hidden chemicals they do not see.

In the end, the story of store-bought fruit finishes at the pie filling and canned fruit aisle. The fruit is coated, colored, preserved, and stickered before your meal. Real fruit's wild side is rejected, but the modified side is a star in every dessert. Sometimes, the only thing truly real is a sticker that nobody meant to eat.

Chapter Eight

Tainted Greens and Fruits, The Grocery's Hidden Dangers

SHOPPING THE PERIMETER OF a grocery store sounds smart for health, but the produce section has its own problems, hidden by fresh colors and perfect shapes. Most vegetables, whether loose, binned, packed, or bagged, are grown using a roster of modern chemicals. Pesticides, herbicides, and fungicides like chlorpyrifos, glyphosate, imidacloprid, fludioxonil, and pyrimethanil are standard. These residues can sink deep into the skin and flesh and do not wash out with water.

If you buy organic, that is better, and later chapters in this book cover organic food fully. Still, studies show more than eighty percent of peaches and cucumbers sampled in U.S. stores carry pesticide residues. Bell peppers, green beans, potatoes, and strawberries are some of the most contaminated vegetables. Even green beans sometimes show banned chemical traces years after they were supposedly removed.

Weeds, bugs, and molds attack crops constantly, so farmers rely on sprays for speed, cost, and big harvests. Celery, for example, is approved for over sixty different pesticides, including methamidophos and maneb, meant to avoid rot and insects, but residues stay.

Pesticides do not just leave after harvest. Chlorpyrifos can damage brains and nerves, especially in kids, and it is banned in the E.U. and highly restricted here. Glyphosate raises questions about cancer, gut trouble, and soil health. Imidacloprid is known for harming pollinators and disrupting ecosystems, and it is commonly found in food. Multiple chemical residues build up in our bodies; the effects do not vanish with a rinse.

Federal standards set by the U.S. EPA are called Maximum Residue Limits. For example, the limit for chlorpyrifos in spinach is 7 parts per million, and for maneb in celery it is 15 ppm. The units used are parts per million for chemicals and becquerels per kilogram for radiation. The U.S. allows levels of pesticide residues five to ten times higher than Europe or Canada, calling them "safe" by American standards.

After the nuclear meltdown in Fukushima, Japan, in March 2011, a radioactive cloud carried isotopes like cesium and iodine that were deposited in rain and dust. This fallout contaminated some fruits, vegetables, and cow's milk in affected regions, especially parts of Japan and areas downwind across the North Pacific. Russia, China, and Vietnam banned food from these areas; the U.S. raised its allowable cesium limit on imported food to 1,200 becquerels per kilogram, twelve times the strict European limit of 100.

Japan itself banned and destroyed foods over 100 becquerels, but America accepted those and more, calling them safe for stores. Nuclear accidents can contaminate soil for decades. You might need to bring a Geiger counter to the store in the future; there are over 450 nuclear power plants active worldwide, plus uranium mines, nuclear bomb test sites, and ongoing leaks.

Some chemical fertilizers add silent dangers. Many contain arsenic, cadmium, and lead. These build up in the soil and plants, affecting carrots, beets, spinach, and beans. Over time, heavy metals hurt the nervous system, kidneys, and bones. Cancer risk goes up after many years of slow, invisible exposure.

Farmers sometimes use untreated or recycled water for irrigation, especially in dry regions. This water can carry pharmaceutical drugs, heavy metals, and antibiotic-resistant bacteria. Cabbage, lettuce, and carrots soak up these substances through the roots. Washing vegetables on the surface will not remove deep residues.

Wind drift spreads chemical sprays beyond targeted fields. People who live near large-scale farms are exposed to drifting pesticide clouds, with health effects ranging from headaches and skin irritation to increased cancer risk and shortened life spans. Nearby organic crops may get ruined by spray drift. Bad manure or contaminated hay can stunt, twist, and even destroy vegetable crops. In recent years, many farms have had sales banned due to high levels of PFAS or heavy metals with no label or warning at the store.

Imported vegetables and fruit raise new questions. Foods come from Mexico, Chile, China, and Southeast Asia. Some banned pesticides include acephate, methamidophos, and DDT. Acephate causes nervous-system symptoms, and DDT is linked to cancer and birth defects. U.S. stores do not list all chemical treatments or clearly show country of origin on mixed items. In theory, bulk mixed vegetables from a poorly regulated country could be sprayed with anything, shipped to the U.S., packed, wholesaled, and distributed without anyone knowing what you eat.

Garlic from China is often reported as grown in untreated human-waste fields. Bulbs can absorb lead, E. coli, and pharmaceuticals, and tests have found high contamination, yet packages rarely warn buyers. Your "fresh" garlic or snap peas may be a lot less safe or natural than they look.

Even locally grown apples are heavily sprayed. In Michigan, orchardists use up to fifty pounds of chemical spray per acre each year, including captan, carbaryl, and glyphosate. Sprays fight worms, scabs, and fungus, but many residues remain on the apples. Apples are also coated in wax containing morpholine. Morpholine can combine with stomach acid and vegetable nitrates to form nitrosamines, a possible cancer risk. If fingerprints stick after washing, the wax is not natural.

Produce is endlessly handled at every step—harvesting, packing, filling, sorting, and display. Each time food is moved, bacteria and viruses hitch a ride. Surveys have found over ninety-nine percent of produce bins and store scales covered with germ colonies. Each touch is another chance for contamination by norovirus, E. coli, mold, or staph.

Precut and pre-washed vegetables are no better. Bagged greens, shredded carrots, and diced peppers travel through many hands and machines. Damp bags let Listeria, Salmonella, and E. coli grow. In 2018, tainted romaine lettuce sickened more than two hundred people in thirty-six states; ninety-six were hospitalized, and five died. Bad irrigation water or a handler not washing hands can start a national outbreak. Triple washing does not always clean every scar or leaf vein.

Bulk bins and deli containers carry risks. Un-sanitized scoops, plastics, and mixed batches can spread germs, mildew, and BPA from old containers. Vegetables moved from old bins to new ones carry invisible risks. Investigators have found Salmonella in many bins after vegetables sat for several days. Washing vegetables helps but will never erase every problem. Chemical residues leach into flesh. Bacteria and molds settle in scars. Even home washing can only reach the surface. Organic produce can also be contaminated by drift, water, or manure gone bad.

Some produce is treated with radiation or X-rays before reaching your cart. Food irradiation kills bugs and bacteria and delays spoilage. U.S. agencies allow it for papaya, mango, guava, and some berries, along with mushrooms, onions, and potatoes. Radiation does not make food radioactive, but it can lower vitamin C and B vitamins and slightly change flavor or texture.

Studies find minor chemical byproducts from irradiation, but the long-term impact is still debated.

Sometimes radiation comes by accident. The world has over 450 active nuclear plants, countless mines, bomb test sites, and leaks. Fallout from disasters can poison farmland for generations. After Fukushima in 2011, Japan banned contaminated food, but America accepted higher radiation levels. A few foods are naturally radioactive—bananas, Brazil nuts, and potatoes carry potassium-40. No one has ever gotten radiation sickness from eating them, but they are a reminder that nature is complicated and the modern supply chain is even more so.

Your "healthy" grocery pile is the result of a global system packed with invisible risks. Unlisted sprays, heavy metals, bacteria from hands, molds, wax, plastics, irradiation, or garlic grown in sewage all show up in your basket. Scrub, peel, and rinse, but know the truth is deeper than the skin. If every vegetable carried a label telling you its story, most shoppers would pause before eating.

Chapter Nine

The Milky Mirage, Poisons in Your Carton

WELL, WE ARE PERIMETER shopping again and now stand in the dairy section. Nothing beats a chill from the cooler and a wall of milk, butter, cheese, and tubs of soft, white stuff. Sadly, the dairy aisle is contaminated, too. It only looks pure and creamy beneath all that bright white and yellow shine.

Milk starts at the cow and her daily feast. Cows eat corn, soy, alfalfa, and cottonseed, much of it sprayed with pesticides such as chlorpyrifos, atrazine, and permethrin. These chemicals kill pests, molds, and weeds, and a portion of that feed story ends up in the milk. Milk carries not only nutrients but a chemical story. Whenever there is a nuclear leak, disaster, or fallout, milk is the first thing tested.

After the Fukushima nuclear meltdown in 2011, the first radioactive food detected in the U.S. was cow milk in Hawaii. Radiation in milk has also been found after Chernobyl and U.S. testing sites, sometimes showing up for years. Many batches go untested, or problems are discovered only after people have already consumed the product.

Even after pasteurization, trace residues sneak into conventional milk. Large national surveys have found pesticide residues in many conventional samples; one study reported chlorpyrifos, atrazine, and permethrin in 26–60% of conventional milk but none in organic. Chlorpyrifos is a nerve poison, banned in the E.U. but still detected in U.S. milk from conventional farms.

It is linked to brain problems in children, memory loss, and headaches. Atrazine and permethrin may act as endocrine disruptors, altering hormones. Research has found higher pesticide residues in milk from regions with heavy chemical farming. Drinking milk with these disruptors has been tied to altered hormone levels, early puberty, smaller birth weight, fertility trouble, and some cancers, with children in farming regions showing more learning issues and lower test scores.

Cows get sick, so farmers use antibiotics—and not all of that stays in the animal. Studies in the U.S. have found residues of common antibiotics in conventional milk, including sulfonamides and beta-lactam drugs; some samples have exceeded federal tolerance limits. These residues contribute to antibiotic resistance, weaken gut bacteria, and can trigger allergic reactions, hives, vomiting, or digestive upset in sensitive children. Repeated exposure can upset the immune system and make vulnerable people more likely to battle persistent infections.

If your immune system is already weak, antibiotic residues can wipe out more of your good gut bacteria. With fewer natural defenses, every glass of milk becomes a new risk, especially for children, the elderly, and those with chronic health issues.

Growth hormones in dairy sit at the center of a health and ethics storm. Many conventional dairy cows receive recombinant Bovine Somatotropin (rBST), also called recombinant Bovine Growth Hormone (rBGH), a lab-made version of a natural cow hormone that controls milk production. It pushes the cow's body to keep giving high volumes of milk long after normal production would slow.

Conventional U.S. milk has been found to contain much higher levels of growth-related hormones than certified organic milk, which bans these injections. That extra hormone load does not stay in the barn; it ends up in the bulk tank and then in your glass. rBGH use is linked to more udder infections in cows, because animals pushed to produce more milk face more stress and inflammation in the udder.

More infections mean more antibiotic treatments, which increases the risk of antibiotic residues and resistant bacteria moving through the food chain. For humans, concern centers on IGF-1 (Insulin-like Growth Factor-1), a powerful growth signal that rises when cows receive these hormones and that can also rise in people who consume large amounts of hormone-treated dairy. Elevated IGF-1 levels have been associated in research with higher risks of certain cancers and with changes in growth and maturation patterns, including earlier puberty in girls.

Canada and the European Union do not allow rbST/rBGH use in dairy herds, citing animal-welfare problems and potential long-term human health effects. Their regulators accept that the hormone injections harm cows and that the added IGF-1 and hormone disturbance may pose unacceptable risks. In contrast, the U.S. still allows these hormones in dairy, and milk from treated cows is mixed into the conventional supply without any requirement to label it. Economic pressure favors higher yield per cow, and industry lobbying has kept these products on the market despite bans overseas.

For shoppers, that leaves a difficult choice. Organic standards prohibit rBST and rBGH, and many smaller dairies advertise that they do not use artificial growth hormones even if they are not fully organic. Cartons that say "from cows not treated with rBST or rBGH" usually reflect a different production philosophy, one that accepts lower yield per cow in exchange for fewer hormones and fewer infections. When you pick up a gallon, you are not only buying milk; you are voting on whether profit or precaution wins in the barns that supply your table.

Milk and cream can also contain heavy metals from irrigation water, farm soil, and cattle feed. Lead, cadmium, arsenic, and mercury can show up in dairy products. These toxic metals weaken bones, strain kidneys, and permanently lower IQ in children. Milk batches with metal contamination sometimes cause recalls or lawsuits.

Toxic mold in the animal's grain and feed brings another invisible hazard. Aflatoxins come from moldy corn or stored grains; their milk metabolite, aflatoxin M1, often enters milk, cheese, and even infant formula. These are potent liver carcinogens, classified by IARC as Group 1 carcinogens and linked to liver cancer, growth stunting, immune suppression, and other chronic damage. Pasteurization does not reliably destroy aflatoxins, so preventing mold in feed is the only real protection.

Most modern feed for dairy cows is genetically engineered, including corn, soy, and alfalfa. The cow's DNA does not change, so the milk itself is not GMO by sequence; still, GMO crops are sprayed with more herbicides and pesticides as weeds and insects evolve to resist chemicals. Residues can concentrate in animal fat and show up in cheese, butter, and yogurt.

Processed dairy foods like cottage cheese, cream cheese, and flavored yogurts often use modified corn starch, thickening gums, or gelatins from GMO sources. These thickeners add texture and shelf life but offer no health benefit. They may trigger gut discomfort, gas, or increase food-allergy risk by altering gut bacteria.

After cows, chemicals, and feed, milk moves on to heat. Pasteurization means heating milk to kill bacteria. Some milk and cream get blasted at ultra-high temperatures for even longer shelf life.

This changes flavor, breaks down proteins, destroys enzymes, and can make it harder for some people to digest. Many children and adults now report milk allergies or lactose intolerance; roughly 20% or more of people have some level of sensitivity, depending on the population.

Modern milk and dairy face a newer threat: microplastics. These are tiny synthetic fibers, flakes, or spheres from plastic equipment or packaging. Independent analyses have found microplastics in powdered milk and in processed cheese and yogurt. Microplastics can cross the gut barrier and may end up in blood, liver, and other tissues. Scientists worry that lifetime exposure could alter hormone levels, damage organs, or interfere with digestion, though long-term data is still being gathered.

What about the color you see? Butter and cheese are often tinted with annatto, turmeric, or synthetic dyes for a stronger yellow or orange. Cheaper cheese uses azo dyes, which are stable but have been linked to allergies and potential cancer concerns in sensitive people. Bright orange cheese or butter does not mean more nutrition; sometimes it means more chemicals.

Next to the butter sit the fake butters and spreads. The ingredient list is long: refined vegetable oils, emulsifiers, colorants, flavorings, and preservatives. These may include trans fats, mono- and diglycerides, and food colorings. The body has no real use for many of these additives. Real butter contains cream and salt; margarine and spreads are food-engineering experiments with unclear long-term health impacts.

Scan the rest of the case. Yogurt, cottage cheese, and sour cream are not safe from extra ingredients. Stabilizers keep them thick and uniform—common ones are guar gum, carrageenan, and modified corn starch, with preservatives added for longer shelf life. Many containers now include corn syrup, artificial sweeteners, and "fruit" made from flavor chemicals and dye. These ingredients feed gut bacteria the wrong way, sometimes causing gas, bloating, or long-term gut trouble.

Americans get more saturated fat from dairy than from almost any other category. Saturated fat, salt, and ultra-processed fillers are top ingredients in cheese, butter, and sour cream. Excess saturated fat is tied to blocked arteries, heart attack, diabetes, and possibly Alzheimer's disease. Many spreads or processed cheese slices now have even less nutrition than a carton of whole milk. The more "convenient" the product, the more likely it is to be high in additives and low in real food value.

Your cheese rarely warns you about extra processing. Mold inhibitors and antifungal preservatives are common, especially in big-brand shredded cheeses. These can cause headaches, digestive stress, or allergy attacks in sensitive people. Some people get skin rashes or asthma from these added preservatives. Yogurt in the United States comes with big promises.

Brands claim gut health or promote extra probiotics, but often offset it with high sugar, fake fruits, and artificial sweeteners. Ground-up imported strawberries or peaches in yogurt can still carry pesticide residues, which pasteurization does not remove.

Too much sugar in yogurt can promote "bad" gut bacteria and gas, driving candida growth rather than a balanced microbiome.

Commercial dairy can go off at any point in the process. If pasteurization, filtration, or refrigeration fails, you can get sick. Cold-chain problems allow milk to grow Salmonella, Listeria, or E. coli before you ever open the carton. Recalls are common; dairy products frequently lead food-recall lists, driven by handling errors and failures at multiple steps.

If you get food poisoning from cheese or milk, it may have started with a small slip in a factory or storage room. None of the risk is isolated. Dairy products stack layers of chemicals, heavy metals, antibiotics, dioxins, pesticides, and drugs like ractopamine. Ractopamine is banned in most countries, including China and much of Europe, but is still approved for some U.S. livestock, contributing residues to the food chain. Dioxins build up over years inside fat and are hard for the body to remove. These industrial residues concentrate in animal fats, making butter, cheese, and whole milk top dietary sources.

With every bite or sip, you are eating from a global supply chain of surprises. Chemicals, contaminants, food colorings, hormones, sweeteners, bacteria, and microplastics are all along for the ride. Next time you see that "all natural" label, look past the marketing. The true story is not in the pretty carton but in the long list of invisible ingredients and treatments. Organic dairy and non-dairy alternatives offer different trade-offs, and those deserve their own chapter. If you think "all natural" is a guarantee, get ready to be surprised.

Buying milk or cheese is no longer a simple act. It takes research, a sense of humor, and some science. Every label is an exercise in trust. Look for shorter ingredient lists, certified organic claims, and farms that test their feed and soil for toxins and metals. If you want purer milk, you now have to hunt for it.

Many readers grew up thinking milk built strong bones and butter meant good health. But the science and food world have changed. Your next glass of milk might be a laboratory experiment with cream on top. The "healthy" dairy aisle now tells a different story, one of chemicals, processing, and risks few consumers truly see. Fewer ingredients, more honest farming, and careful handling are the cure. If only we really got that in every scoop or sip.

Chapter Ten

Sick by the Slice, The Bread That Breaks Our Bodies

Stores display endless aisles of bread, crackers, cookies, cereal, and pasta while people consume wheat daily without questioning its origin. Unlike traditional fields, today's grain is manipulated through intensive breeding and, in some cases, genetic modification to maximize yield, corporate profit, and efficiency. Scientists work on wheat in laboratories to develop "super crops" and faster production, while regulators approve new varieties without long-term health studies for everyday eaters.

Modern grain is engineered to resist disease, stand strong, and withstand harsh weather through chemical treatments, gamma irradiation, and complex breeding programs. Gene-edited strains are tested for disease resistance and baking quality, yet new products often reach the market before anyone has studied their effects over decades of daily use. People rarely associate bread consumption with health issues because they rarely question the origin or safety of the grain they eat each day.

Wheat fields are sprayed with glyphosate, one of the most widely used herbicides in modern agriculture. Glyphosate is toxic to plants and can leave residues in food. Animal and lab studies link glyphosate residues to disruption of gut bacteria, potential immune changes, and concerns about cancer and endocrine effects. Observational research has also associated glyphosate use with higher rates of some cancers, birth outcomes, and kidney problems in exposed communities.

Pesticide exposure is not just about weeds and bugs. Residues can harm developing babies, lower IQ in children, delay development, and make diabetes more likely according to multiple pesticide-health studies. Long-term exposure has been associated with organ damage, memory loss, insulin resistance, and mood changes. Some fields use chemicals that remain detectable in wheat products even after baking.

After harvest, wheat becomes more vulnerable to chemical abuse. Industrial milling crushes, grinds, and heats wheat until most of the bran and germ are stripped away. White flour is left, almost pure starch. This flour is then bleached with chlorine dioxide or benzoyl peroxide, and potassium bromate is used in some brands as a dough improver. Potassium bromate is banned in the European Union, Canada, Brazil, China, India, and many other countries because it is classified as "possibly carcinogenic to humans" and linked to kidney and thyroid damage in animal studies. Yet it still appears in some U.S. breads and rolls.

Bread factories mix flour and additives in large vats, add preservatives, and ship frozen dough nationwide. Local bakeries often bake this frozen dough as "fresh" bread. Antimold agents such as calcium propionate and propionic acid are added to keep bread soft for weeks. These ingredients are linked in sensitive people to migraines, hyperactivity, skin rashes, and gastrointestinal upset. Bread "improvers" aid factory production but add no nutrition.

Dough conditioners and flavor enhancers are common in commercial breads. L-cysteine, often made from human hair or feathers, shortens mixing times and softens dough. Azodicarbonamide is used to bleach or condition flour, but it is banned in some countries due to links to asthma and potential cancer concerns. Mono- and diglycerides are emulsifiers derived from vegetable oils or animal fats; they extend shelf life but may raise blood fat levels and promote inflammation.

Pesticides and natural toxins can stick around in wheat products even after high-heat baking. Flour silos and storage bins may harbor mold or mycotoxins. Aflatoxins from Aspergillus molds are dangerous and can survive the baking process; they are potent liver toxins and recognized liver-cancer risks. Bread sold in grocery stores is often stripped of its natural nutrients. White flour loses most of its fiber, vitamins, minerals, and healthy fats in milling. Companies "enrich" flour with synthetic vitamins, but these do not recreate the whole-grain package. White bread is digested faster than many candy bars, causing blood sugar spikes that trigger hunger.

Most processed wheat products—white bread, buns, pizza, pasta, cookies, cakes, and crackers contain added sugar or corn syrup to boost taste and shelf appeal. Sugar and refined starch digest quickly, driving rapid insulin spikes and feeding belly fat. This blood-sugar rollercoaster tires your pancreas and raises the risk of diabetes and obesity.

Children who eat more processed bread and wheat-based foods show higher rates of fatty liver disease and metabolic syndrome. Metabolic syndrome a cluster of belly fat, high blood pressure, high blood sugar, and abnormal cholesterol sets the stage for diabetes, heart attack, and stroke later in life. These diets often lack fiber and essential nutrients, increasing the risk of digestive upset and inflammation. Wheat-driven insulin resistance throws the body's hormone system off balance and worsens chronic inflammation, which is now tied to conditions like arthritis, dementia, and cancer.

Newer grain varieties contain more gluten than many older crops used for traditional baking. Gluten helps dough rise and gives bread its chewy texture, which most people enjoy. Unfortunately, higher gluten content also makes digestion harder and can increase inflammation in sensitive individuals who eat it regularly. Many people report rashes, headaches, stomach pain, and mood swings after eating baked goods even without a formal diagnosis of celiac disease.

Bread dough and commercial baked goods often use instant yeast, which accelerates rising and reduces factory time. These yeasts can be harder to digest for some people, leading to bloating and gas. Sourdough is typically easier to digest because fermentation helps break down gluten and creates natural acids and preservatives. Industrial yeast lacks these benefits and is bred to be consistent and fast, not gentle on sensitive guts.

Preservatives in wheat products include calcium propionate, potassium sorbate, and, in some cases, sulfites. People report gut pain or headaches from these, including children with asthma or allergies. Additives like cellulose gum, xanthan gum, and guar gum are used to thicken or stabilize mass-produced bread, pasta, and tortillas. Many people notice digestive trouble or feel that these gum-laden foods interfere with normal digestion and possibly vitamin absorption.

Most people assume whole-grain bread is healthy, yet commercial loaves often contain as many artificial additives as refined varieties. For national brands, labels rarely reveal the full story of milling quality or chemical residues, even after baking and packaging. Studies show that many flour-based products test positive for pesticide traces that survive heating during everyday bread production. Children are especially vulnerable, because their smaller bodies absorb toxins more quickly, leading to greater long-term health and developmental risks.

Frequent consumption of refined grain products almost guarantees weight gain for most people because digestion rapidly converts starch into sugar, which drives hunger and overeating. Aggressive snack marketing fuels cycles of over-consumption and nutrient deficiency, leaving people tired yet still craving more processed breads and pastries. What looks wholesome on store shelves often provides few vitamins and far more synthetic ingredients than genuine, whole foods. This pattern contributes to metabolic imbalance and makes preventable diseases increasingly common across industrial food cultures.

Store-bought "fiber" in bread often comes from additives like inulin rather than genuine bran from whole grains, which better support gut health and balance. Such substitutions inflate nutrition labels while offering limited real benefit to digestion or blood-sugar control. Processor shortcuts replace nourishment with filler compounds used to improve texture, appearance, and shelf stability in modern convenience foods. Fast foods and packaged pastries supply dense calories without micronutrients, leaving consumers undernourished despite high energy intake.

Grain crops used for staple foods have become central to the Western diet, contributing to trends in diabetes, dementia, heart disease, and some cancers. Global research links higher intake of refined grain products with obesity and chronic inflammation across generations. True reform would mean replacing industrial flour systems with diverse heritage crops grown under regenerative, low-chemical farming practices. Ultimately, wheat represents both human ingenuity and industrial excess, and the balance between the two will determine whether future diets heal or harm society.

When you reach for bread at the store, pause to ask what is inside. Wheat's long trip from lab to loaf is not a simple one. Food made to last for weeks in a bag often lingers in your body in all the wrong ways. Your favorite sandwich or toast carries more chemical baggage than you ever expected. The story of wheat is a warning against trusting modern grocery shelves more than nature itself.

Chapter Eleven

Sweeteners and Sugar (includes high-fructose corn syrup, sugar alcohols, artificial sweeteners, hidden sugars, metabolic and brain effects)

WALK THROUGH ANY GROCERY aisle, and sweetness appears everywhere in drinks, bread, sauces, snacks, desserts, and even frozen dinners. When a label claims to be free from added sugar, it often replaces it with synthetic syrups and refined chemical substitutes. Companies continually replace natural ingredients with artificial sweeteners, altering taste and health under bright packaging and misleading marketing claims. Almost every packaged product contains traces of syrups, glucose, or engineered compounds that mimic sugar.

In processed foods, the sweetness cycle never stops as manufacturers rely on cane, beet, and corn derivatives in endless formulations. Dozens of extracts, including maltose, dextrose, and chemical syrups, help maintain flavor and keep consumers loyal to consistent in store textures. Sugar substitutes like xylitol, erythritol, and sorbitol fill diet shelves, promising better choices while still tricking taste buds into craving more. Even natural sounding options, such as fruit or plant extracts, become refined products of industrial food science rather than real nourishment.

Honey scandals now expose imitation blends in which rice or corn syrup replaces authentic nectar in many supermarket jars, making honey one of the most frequently adulterated foods in the world. Some brands mix real honey with sweet syrup and sell it as pure, misleading buyers into trusting fake golden liquid as a source of nutrition. Imported blends often carry labels like wildflower, though they lack the minerals, enzymes, and pollen vital for genuine bee sourced benefits. Local beekeepers are more likely to maintain integrity by producing uncut honey naturally rich in micronutrients, which are otherwise stripped during bulk refining and ultra filtering.

Modern labels promising zero sugar or sugar free often hide chemical replacements that appear in everyday meals and are marketed as healthy convenience. Common staples, including cereal, bread, yogurt, and protein bars, now rely on engineered sweetness to extend shelf life and drive sales. Consumers rarely recognize the many names scattered across ingredient lists, even though regulators track dozens of different sweeteners and sugar forms in their databases. In truth, both added sugar and imitation formulas sustain the same dependence cycle that began with sugar itself.

The food industry plays a long game with lab sweeteners. In the 1970s, saccharin, cyclamate, and later aspartame hit mainstream markets, each bringing safety questions and, at times, bans or warnings from regulators after animal studies suggested possible cancer risks. The approval process for artificial sweeteners has been among the most contested in FDA history, with criticism over conflicts of interest and heavy reliance on industry funded research while independent findings of harm were often downplayed. Today, compounds like aspartame, acesulfame potassium, and sucralose appear in diet soda, yogurt, gum, and vitamins despite ongoing debate about their long term safety.

Real sugar from cane is no bargain either. Cane stalks are crushed, juiced, clarified, boiled, spun in a centrifuge, filtered, and dried into granules. Refining steps such as carbonation, filtration, and bleaching strip away all plant fiber and natural micronutrients. All you are left with is almost pure sucrose, an empty carbohydrate, a factory product with more in common with industrial input than with fruit or honey.

In our bodies, these sweeteners cause real trouble. Sugar and syrup overload cells, cause insulin spikes, force the liver to store fat, and drive inflammation throughout the body. Type 2 diabetes, obesity, and non alcoholic fatty liver disease are sweeping the United States and much of the world, with added sugars playing a major role. More than 37 million Americans have diabetes, and many more have prediabetes, while NAFLD affects roughly a quarter of U.S. adults and obesity rates exceed 40 percent.

Most chronic diseases today owe something to sugar or fake sweeteners. Blood pressure climbs, arteries stiffen, cancer risk rises, and cell damage builds up. Large studies show that high added sugar intake from soft drinks, desserts, and processed foods is associated with higher death rates from heart disease and other causes. One analysis estimated that sugary drinks contribute to well over one hundred thousand deaths per year worldwide from diabetes and cardiovascular disease.

The link between sweeteners and sickness does not stop with obesity or diabetes. Sugar and its chemical copies spark chronic inflammation, the hidden fire behind heart disease, some cancers, and many autoimmune and pain conditions. High sugar intake is tied to worse arthritis, more frequent migraines, mood swings, fatigue, and flare ups of inflammatory bowel and skin disorders in many people. Patients often receive drugs for pain or inflammation while the real driver is blood sugar swings and the supercharged level of sweetness in the modern diet.

Artificial sweeteners carry their own risks. They may seem diet friendly, but long term studies suggest they are not a free pass. Observational research ties higher intakes of non caloric sweeteners and diet soft drinks to headaches, weight gain, more belly fat, higher rates of metabolic syndrome, and increased risks of heart attacks, strokes, and overall cardiovascular disease. Some studies also report links with dementia and faster cognitive decline, though debate continues about mechanisms. These chemicals can disrupt gut bacteria, worsen appetite control, alter hormone signals, and may promote fat storage instead of helping with weight loss. Many regular diet drinkers end up heavier and sicker than people who mainly drink water.

Check any random label and you will find sweeteners where you least expect them, in bread, sauces, drinks, yogurt, and protein snacks. A single can of cola typically contains around 35 to 40 grams of added sugar, roughly the total daily limit many guidelines recommend not exceeding, and ice cream or cereal bars can add even more. Manufacturers sweeten daily foods to keep consumers craving more through repeated bursts of quick energy and familiar addictive taste profiles. Those small daily choices build habits far stronger than people realize, shaping weight, mood, and long term health.

Labeling systems make it challenging to avoid hidden sweetness because sweeteners appear under dozens of names that few shoppers recognize. Terms such as agave syrup, malt extract, evaporated cane juice, brown rice syrup, or fruit juice concentrate can mislead buyers who think they are choosing natural products. Public health agencies note that there are more than 60 common names for added sugars alone, not counting artificial sweeteners and sugar alcohols, and many are buried in long multisyllabic words on colorful packaging. If you cannot pronounce a sweetening additive, there is a good chance it is a refined compound designed to mimic the body's response to sugar.

Laboratory sweeteners promise low or zero calories but bring new problems because they depend on chemical reactions, acids, and stabilizers used in mass production. Some blends can leave traces of solvents or reaction byproducts that the liver must process along with the sweetener itself. Experts caution that not all replacements deliver the intended diet benefits and that risk may increase with repeated long term consumption, especially when these products also contain dyes, preservatives, and emulsifiers. Industrial formulations prioritize color and texture over nutrition, turning modern treats into chemistry projects disguised as safe indulgences.

Once digested, both added sugars and artificial sweeteners alter blood sugar rhythms and strain organs responsible for regulating glucose, appetite, and metabolism, locking people into daily cycles of craving and fatigue. These same compounds can disrupt healthy gut bacteria, leading to bloating, fatigue, and poor nutrient absorption among frequent consumers of processed foods. Research shows that microbiome imbalances can alter mood, immunity, and digestion throughout the body more quickly than once believed, so a sweetened diet is not just about weight but about whole body balance.

The health effects of chronic sweetener use are visible everywhere. Insulin resistance, non alcoholic fatty liver, high blood pressure, constant hunger, and brain fog trace back to excess sugar and fake sugar in many lives. Childhood obesity has more than doubled in recent decades, and nearly one in five U.S. children now meets criteria for obesity, with sugary snacks, sports drinks, breakfast bars, and fruit flavored gummies helping drive disease before adulthood even begins. Sweet foods strip minerals, weaken bones and teeth, and trigger hidden inflammation that can fuel chronic pain, muscle aches, joint stiffness, and autoimmune flares over a lifetime.

The marketing engine never stops moving, covering unhealthy realities with comforting words like natural, organic, pure, or wholesome on every label. Packages often promise purity while hiding processed stevia, monk fruit extract, maltitol, agave syrup, or brown rice sweeteners in the fine print. Reading ingredient lists becomes a chemistry lesson filled with long words and complex blends disguised as natural sources of flavor and texture.

If the label lists many different sweeteners or confusing scientific names, it is a warning sign. Companies rename syrups and sweet compounds using terms such as fructose, dextrose, glucose solids, or concentrated fruit juices that keep consumers guessing about what they are really eating. Crystalline blends and concentrated juices look harmless but deliver much the same metabolic burden now associated with sugar.

Solutions are possible. Cooking at home more often, reading every label, and refusing products with multiple hidden sweeteners are powerful steps. Choosing small amounts of local honey, real maple syrup, and whole fruit instead of industrial sweeteners helps lower the total sugar load. Drinking water or herbal tea and retraining your taste buds to appreciate plain, unsweetened food can gradually break dependence on constant sweetness. Studies show that cutting back on added sugar can improve energy, reduce brain fog, support weight loss, and ease joint and muscle pain within weeks as blood sugar and inflammation begin to settle.

Newer sweeteners are largely creations of scientists, not gifts from nature. Childhood obesity, diabetes, low energy, weak immunity, and chronic pain are part of the price society pays for eating lab made sweet in nearly every meal and snack. Real food does not need sugar in every bite or sip. Even one week with far less sweetness can start to improve how you feel. The true taste of real food may surprise you, and you may no longer crave the packaged, sweetened cycle once your body remembers what normal feels like.

Chapter Twelve

Bakery and Ready-to-Eat Foods with International & Ethnic Foods (covering pastries, sweets, in-store bakery, imported snacks and bakery items, specialty sweets, and ingredient risks worldwide)

Most store bought pastries bypass traditional craftsmanship entirely. Frozen dough arrives pre formed in trucks, where chemical stabilizers and emulsifiers extend shelf life dramatically. Commercial bakeries rely heavily on additives like xanthan gum, guar gum, and mono and diglycerides to control moisture, improve texture, and keep products on shelves longer. Pepperidge Farm frozen puff pastry squares, a standard in many bakeries, contain enriched wheat flour, water, vegetable oils such as palm, soybean, and hydrogenated cottonseed, high fructose corn syrup, salt, mono and diglycerides, soy lecithin, and malted barley flour. Each dough piece can remain stable for months at low freezer temperatures, then thaw and bake into what customers perceive as fresh baked.

In store cupcakes are decorated with industrial icings loaded with artificial colors and concentrated sugars. A typical medium bakery cupcake contains roughly 350 to 450 calories and about 25 to 40 grams of added sugar, depending on flavor. For context, the American Heart Association recommends no more than 25 grams of added sugar per day for most women and 36 grams for most men, so one cupcake can use or exceed the entire daily allowance. Halloween candy surveys have identified products like candy corn and brightly colored gummies that still contain Red Dye 3, a color linked to cancer in animal tests and banned from cosmetics since 1990 yet still allowed in some foods in the United States.

Dunkin Donuts style glazed and powdered donuts use commercial formulations built for softness and shelf life, based on enriched wheat flour, sugar, modified starches, and emulsifiers like DATEM and monoglycerides to strengthen dough and keep it tender. Ingredient lists also often include artificial flavors, soy lecithin, color agents such as titanium dioxide, and preservatives like potassium sorbate and sodium benzoate so the donuts stay fresh tasting longer.

Muffins are essentially cakes in disguise and often surpass cheeseburgers in sugar load. A jumbo muffin from a chain bakery can reach about 540 to 680 calories with more than 40 grams of sugar per serving, while coffee shop scones that look simpler usually include flour, sugar, leavening agents, fat, and milk as a base plus commercial preservatives and artificial flavors. Chain style scones and muffins frequently contain multiple emulsifiers and stabilizers that never appear on the menu board.

International bakery goods carry added risks from imported ingredients. In 2023, the FDA recalled several cinnamon applesauce products after finding high lead levels tied to contaminated cinnamon processed abroad, and by early 2024 hundreds of U.S. children across dozens of states had elevated blood lead levels from these snacks. Independent testing has also detected concerning levels of heavy metals such as lead and cadmium in some popular chocolate brands sold in the United States. A festival sweet made with imported milk powder, nuts, and colorings can easily become a chemical stew, with pesticide residues, heavy metals, and restricted dyes all present in a single bite yet almost impossible for the consumer to trace.

Azo dyes represent a class of synthetic food colorings that can break down into aromatic amines, some of which raise toxicity concerns. European regulators require warning labels or strict limits for certain azo dyes because of evidence linking them with hyperactivity and behavior changes in some children. Approved dyes there, such as Sunset Yellow, Azorubine, Amaranth, and Allura Red, still appear widely in U.S. pastries, candies, and festival treats but without the same warnings.

Food scandals in sweets are not hypothetical. In 2008, more than 50,000 infants in China became ill and several died after consuming formula adulterated with melamine, a nitrogen rich chemical that falsely boosted measured protein content but caused kidney stones and kidney failure. Subsequent U.S. testing found melamine and related compounds in imported candies, cookies, and milk based snacks that used contaminated ingredients. When milk powder from a facility with past melamine issues meets nuts with undeclared pesticide residues and colorants restricted overseas, a single pastry can layer multiple hazards that no single inspection catches.

Titanium dioxide is widely used to whiten and brighten pastries, frostings, and donuts to create the pristine look customers expect. In 2021, the European Food Safety Authority concluded that genotoxicity for titanium dioxide particles could not be ruled out, because they can cause DNA and chromosome damage in laboratory studies, and France banned its use in food earlier. Animal research has shown intestinal inflammation and precancerous changes in rats fed titanium dioxide, and more recent cell studies report DNA damage and raise concern about long term cancer risk, especially from nanoparticle forms. Despite these red flags, titanium dioxide remains permitted in many U.S. baked goods and icings.

Many supposedly wholesome oat cookies and cream filled pastries contain propylene glycol and mono and diglycerides to keep them soft for weeks without refrigeration. Propylene glycol acts as a solvent and texture agent and is generally recognized as safe at low levels, but high or chronic intake can pose risks for people with kidney or liver problems because they cannot clear it efficiently. Experimental work suggests propylene glycol and similar agents can increase intestinal permeability, which may worsen symptoms in people with inflammatory or autoimmune gut conditions. Yet cumulative exposure for heavy consumers of packaged baked goods has not been well studied.

Festival food vendors and farmers market sellers often operate with less oversight than licensed plants. Trays of powdered sugar donuts, pastries, or baklava laid out on open tables usually lack ingredient labels, allergen warnings, or lot codes. Open display invites cross contamination and temperature abuse, and outbreak investigations have traced pathogens such as E coli, Listeria, and Salmonella to festival and imported sweets. In 2025, for example, investigators linked an outbreak of Salmonella infections in several states to mini pastries produced in Italy and distributed through a U.S. warehouse, with laboratory tests confirming contamination in product samples.

Food allergy incidents underline the stakes. In one well documented case, a wedding guest with a severe nut allergy developed anaphylaxis after a caterer who had promised nut free food served items that contained undeclared nuts. More recently, federal alerts have highlighted recalls of mixed nut products for undeclared hazelnuts, and regulators warn that individuals with hazelnut allergy face a risk of serious or life threatening reactions if exposed. When pastries and sweets are sold without clear ingredient and allergen labeling, each bite becomes a gamble for sensitive people.

Even specialty holiday sweets have drawn regulatory attention. Some Chinese style mooncakes sold in North America have tested positive for sodium dehydroacetate, a preservative banned from certain traditional products in China after authorities raised concerns about liver and kidney toxicity from long term intake. Inspections have also found mooncake brands that used egg wash but failed to declare egg as an allergen on packaging, leaving people with egg allergies unaware of the risk.

The recall record for baked goods keeps growing. In mid 2025, more than two million pastries and related products were recalled in the United States and Canada over potential Listeria contamination, affecting dozens of product types and long distribution chains. Separate investigations that year documented at least one Salmonella outbreak tied to imported pastries, with confirmed illnesses across multiple states. These events show how easily contamination in one bakery or plant can travel nationwide.

Cream horns and eclairs often rely on hydrogenated vegetable oils to maintain crisp shells and stable fillings over long shelf lives. A commercial sugar coated cream horn can sit at room temperature for many months without spoiling. The pastry dough typically combines hydrogenated fats with synthetic vanilla made from petroleum derived or wood based vanillin, plus emulsifiers and stabilizers. These products are engineered for stability and profit, not nutrition, concentrating refined fats, sugars, and flavor chemicals into a long lasting, low value food.

The safest path for bakery and sweet consumption requires vigilance. Choose treats with short, clear labels listing ingredients you recognize and can pronounce. Avoid unlabeled festival treats and rainbow colored sweets that lack full ingredient and allergen information. When in doubt, ask bakers or vendors directly about dyes, preservatives, and allergens, and treat hesitation or vague answers as a red flag.

For those who love pastries, baking at home with a handful of basic ingredients such as flour, butter, eggs, sugar, vanilla, baking powder, and salt avoids many industrial additives, including titanium dioxide, propylene glycol, and synthetic dyes. When seeking international or specialty flavors, look for certified facilities with transparent sourcing and a track record of meeting FDA or equivalent standards, rather than unregistered kitchens or open air stalls. The best pastries and sweets deserve appreciation, but the industrial versions packed with chemical risks deserve healthy skepticism every time they land on your plate.

Chapter Thirteen

Cooking Oils and Fats

EVERYWHERE YOU LOOK IN the grocery store, you see oils and fats. They are not just in bottles of corn oil, canola oil, or vegetable oil, but hidden deep inside crackers, chips, bread, frozen pizza, and ready made salads. Most people use these oils every day, not realizing they can harm the body at many steps.

Modern cooking oils mostly come from seeds, not olives or coconuts. Many bottles start with industrial crops such as soybeans, canola, corn, sunflower, safflower, cottonseed, and grapeseed, often grown with intensive chemicals and, in the case of soy and corn, frequently from genetically engineered varieties. The seeds are crushed and typically extracted with solvents like hexane to pull out as much oil as possible. Hexane is a petroleum derived chemical used as an industrial solvent; it is later removed by heating and steam, but trace residues can remain at low levels. The crude oil is then refined, bleached, and deodorized to remove color, flavor, and odors. This high level of processing strips out most natural compounds such as vitamin E and many antioxidants, leaving a nearly pure fat that bears little resemblance to the original seed.

Oils that are cheap, clear, and almost flavorless have spent much of their life in refineries. The human body did not evolve on these highly refined, chemically treated fats, and diets very high in them are linked to fatty liver, insulin resistance, and metabolic trouble, especially when they come packaged in ultra processed foods. Our digestive enzymes can technically break them down, but when these oils dominate the diet and displace whole foods, many people develop sluggish digestion, chronic fatigue, and blood lipid problems over time.

Hydrogenation is another factory trick. Liquid oils are partially hardened to make margarine, shortening, and some shelf stable snack fats by reacting them with hydrogen at high temperature in the presence of metal catalysts. This process can create trans fats, which raise LDL cholesterol, lower HDL cholesterol, and increase inflammation, sharply elevating the risk of heart attack and stroke. Because of this, industrial trans fats have been banned or essentially eliminated in the European Union, Canada, and many other countries, and the U.S. has largely removed partially hydrogenated oils from the food supply, though small amounts of trans fat can still appear from high heat processing or labeling loopholes.

To get around trans fat bans, manufacturers increasingly turn to interesterified fats. These are made by rearranging fatty acids on the glycerol backbone using enzymes or chemical catalysts to create customized melting properties for spreads, frostings, and bakery fillings. Early research suggests some interesterified fats may worsen blood lipids, raise fasting blood sugar, and increase inflammatory markers compared with more natural fats, but long term human data remain limited and not reassuring.

Seed oils are naturally high in omega 6 fats, especially linoleic acid. Small amounts are essential, but modern diets in the United States and other industrial countries supply very high omega 6 intake and relatively little omega 3 from fish and certain plant foods. Estimates suggest many people now consume 10 to 20 times more omega 6 than omega 3, while traditional diets likely had ratios closer to 1 to 1 or 2 to 1. This skewed balance is associated with higher chronic inflammation and has been linked to heart disease, arthritis, obesity, diabetes, and some cancers in observational and mechanistic studies. Simply swapping animal fat for large amounts of refined seed oil does not reliably improve inflammation or cardiovascular outcomes and may worsen lipid and metabolic profiles when done in the context of ultra processed diets.

Heating these oils at high temperatures adds another layer of risk. Refined oils have specific smoke points, but even below visible smoking they begin to oxidize and break down into reactive compounds. Deep frying and repeated heating of vegetable oils produces aldehydes and other oxidation products that can damage DNA and proteins, contribute to atherosclerosis, and may increase cancer risk. Restaurants and fast food outlets often reuse fryer oil for long periods, and the longer oil is held at high heat, the more degradation products accumulate. Each batch of fries, nuggets, or onion rings carries not only fat but a load of oxidized byproducts formed in the fryer.

Frozen and processed fried foods are part of the same problem. Many par fried items in the freezer case are pre cooked in large industrial fryers filled with refined oils that are used over and over before the food is flash frozen and shipped. Consumers have no way to know how long that oil was used or how degraded it became during production. Refining and bleaching steps can also form contaminants called 3 MCPD and glycidyl esters in certain refined oils, especially palm based products, and these compounds have been linked to kidney toxicity and potential cancer risks in animal studies.

Preservatives such as BHA, BHT, and TBHQ are commonly added to bottled oils, crackers, cereals, and chips to slow rancidity. These synthetic antioxidants help stop fats from oxidizing on the shelf, but BHA and BHT are considered possible carcinogens in some evaluations and have shown endocrine and allergy related effects in animal studies. Several countries, including some in Europe and Japan, restrict or discourage their use, yet they remain permitted in many U.S. foods. TBHQ, another fat preservative, is also used in industrial products like varnishes; high doses in animal studies have been tied to immune and neurobehavioral changes, though typical food exposures are lower.

Light, air, and time further damage stored oils. Clear plastic bottles on warm, bright shelves allow light and oxygen to accelerate oxidation even before cooking begins. Rancid oil develops off flavors and odors and can cause nausea or digestive upset, but even mildly oxidized oil that still tastes acceptable contains breakdown products that are stressful for the gut and liver to handle. Meanwhile, recent research has detected microplastic particles in many edible oils, likely leaching in from plastic packaging and processing equipment, adding another contaminant load.

Our bodies can handle reasonable amounts of natural fats, but diets built on industrial oils and deep fried foods strain digestion, bile production, and liver detoxification. Many people with high intakes of fried fast food and packaged snacks report chronic bloating, gallbladder trouble, unexplained abdominal pain, and persistent fatigue. Fat accumulation in the liver is now extremely common and is strongly associated with high intakes of refined fats and sugars together, the hallmark of modern processed diets.

Deep fried fast food is the disaster at the end of the oil pipeline. In many kitchens, oil is heated all day, cooled, filtered, and reheated, creating a stew of oxidized fats and frying byproducts. Neither straining nor topping up with fresh oil fully reverses this damage. Each order of fries, chicken pieces, or battered snacks absorbs some of this altered oil, delivering a mixture of unstable fats and aldehydes that no human cells can use constructively. Children and pregnant women are especially vulnerable, because developing organs and brains are more sensitive to oxidative and endocrine disruption, and detoxification systems are not fully robust.

Most ready made salad dressings, mayonnaise, frozen meals, pizzas, boxed cakes, microwave dinners, and instant noodles rely on refined seed oils as major ingredients. Choosing gluten free or even some organic processed products does not necessarily avoid these fats, because they are used for texture and shelf stability across categories. Marketing terms like heart healthy are often applied to vegetable oils based solely on cholesterol lowering potential, but large reviews show that focusing only on cholesterol while ignoring oxidation, ultra processing, and overall diet pattern can be misleading, and replacing traditional foods with high omega 6 refined oils has not eliminated heart disease.

What should you do instead? Traditional fats like butter, ghee, and extra virgin olive oil, used in moderate amounts, are generally easier to digest and bring natural antioxidants and fat soluble nutrients. Avocado oil and coconut oil can also be reasonable options for many people when minimally processed. Whole foods such as fatty fish, nuts, seeds, and high quality animal fats from well raised animals provide more balanced fatty acid profiles and important fat soluble vitamins, rather than the stripped down calories from refined seed oils.

To cut risk, limit ultra processed foods and focus on cooking at home. Buy smaller bottles of real, minimally refined oils you can use within a couple of months, choose glass over plastic when possible, and store oils in dark, cool places. Cook at moderate temperatures, use gentler methods like steaming, stewing, roasting, or baking instead of frequent deep frying, and be cautious with restaurant fried foods where oil age is unknown. Labels that brag about being cholesterol free or light on oil are often just marketing; margarine and many spreads add industrial complexity without proven health benefit.

Watch for hidden oils in bars, granola, crackers, and microwave snacks, where ingredient lists often reveal multiple different seed oils used solely to extend shelf life. Human physiology did not develop on this tide of chemically processed oil, and the global rise in heart disease, stroke, diabetes, and fatty liver has tracked closely with the spread of ultra processed, seed oil heavy diets.

Reducing these oils and choosing simpler, traditional fats can support almost every part of health. Many people notice less joint pain, steadier energy, better digestion, and improved blood markers after shifting away from industrial oils toward real, whole foods. Even a short trial eating without most seed oils and deep fried items can reveal how different the body feels. Once you see and feel the difference, choosing fats that nature made rather than what factories engineered becomes much easier.

Chapter Fourteen

Coffee, Tea, and Beverages (bottled drinks, soda, energy drinks, caffeine, additives, plastic/metal contamination)

COFFEE, TEA, AND BOTTLED drinks are everywhere in the grocery store. They fill aisles, coolers, and checkout shelves, and most of them contain far more than water, leaves, or beans. What you see on the label is only a small part of what is really inside.

Most drinks start far away, on coffee or tea plantations sprayed with pesticides, fungicides, and herbicides. Studies show that imported teas, especially from parts of China, India, and Southeast Asia, often carry measurable pesticide residues, sometimes above local limits, and many samples also contain detectable levels of heavy metals such as lead, arsenic, cadmium, and mercury. These metals accumulate from polluted soil, industrial runoff, and emissions from mines, smelters, and factories and can build up in leaves and beans over years, especially in regions with poor environmental controls.

Heavy metals do not vanish when tea is brewed or coffee is instantized. Reviews of brewed teas have found that a large share of samples steeped for just a few minutes still contained enough lead to raise concern for pregnant women, and instant coffee products in some surveys contained cadmium, lead, nickel, zinc, chromium, and arsenic in more than half the brands tested. Mycotoxins, toxic compounds made by molds that grow on damp or poorly stored beans and leaves, add another invisible risk, damaging cells, straining the liver and kidneys, and contributing to symptoms such as headaches, nausea, and brain fog. The risk is highest in humid climates, where storage and shipping conditions are harder to control.

Water quality at the point of production matters too. In many developing regions, water used to wash, rinse, or brew teas and coffees can carry bacteria, parasites, industrial chemicals, or metals, and leaves or beans may take up some of these contaminants. Boiling kills many microbes but does not remove heavy metals, pesticide residues, or most chemical pollutants, so poor processing and weak safety testing can multiply the risks long before a drink reaches a bottle or bag.

During processing, more chemicals often join the mix. Beans or leaves may be dried, smoked, artificially flavored, sprayed with preservatives, or fermented in ways that can also increase mycotoxin levels if quality is poor. Single serve plastic coffee pods have been shown to leach phthalates and other plasticizers into hot drinks; these chemicals can disrupt hormones and are not nutrients the body expects. Decaffeinated coffee usually requires solvents, and one common solvent, methylene chloride, is approved at low levels but is also classified as a probable carcinogen and suspected reproductive toxin, meaning even trace contamination remains controversial.

Roasting adds another layer. When coffee beans or cereal grains are roasted to medium or dark levels, they form acrylamide, a probable human carcinogen that has caused nerve and DNA damage in animal studies. Acrylamide arises whenever certain amino acids and sugars are heated to high temperatures, so brewed coffee, instant coffee, roasted grain beverages, and chicory blends all contain some amount, with darker roasts and instant products sometimes testing higher.

Factory hygiene and cleaning practices can add yet more residues. Industrial beverage plants must sanitize tanks, pipes, and fillers, but cheap detergents, bleaches, and drying agents are not always fully rinsed away, especially in low cost operations. Over time, plastic hoses, seals, and gaskets can shed microplastics and chemical additives into drinks, and flavor or color changes after long storage hint at oxidation and chemical breakdown inside the sealed bottle or can. Cross contamination is common: the same lines often handle products with nuts, milk powder, soy, gluten grains, or other allergens, so people have suffered allergic reactions to "pure" herbal teas that actually carried traces of peanut or tree nut protcins.

Bulk and cheap teas often contain more than leaves. Some blends include stems, dust, low grade particles, or off label plant material that would not qualify as food in stricter systems, and tests have found so called herbal or slimming teas containing undeclared prescription drugs and stimulants. This means a person drinking what appears to be a natural detox tea could unknowingly ingest pharmaceutical agents that affect heart rate, blood pressure, or mood.

Packaging introduces its own hazards. Many bottled drinks use PET plastic, which is rated for single, cold use but can leach antimony, plasticizers, and other chemicals into the liquid, especially when bottles are stored in hot cars, bright sun, or warehouses without climate control. Acidic drinks such as soda, flavored waters, and bottled teas can pull more of these chemicals out of plastic and linings over time. Even "BPA free" plastic bottles and can liners often use related bisphenols or epoxies that may have similar hormone disrupting effects but have not been thoroughly tested.

Aluminum cans rely on epoxy or similar linings to keep contents from corroding the metal. With time, acid and heat help these linings shed microscopic fragments and molecules into the drink, and products stored warm or for months at a time accumulate more of this chemical load. Shipping and storage make all of this worse, because temperature swings and long warehouse stays accelerate breakdown of plastics, sweeteners, flavors, and colorings in bottles and cans.

To keep drinks shelf stable, bottlers and manufacturers add preservatives such as sodium benzoate, potassium sorbate, and EDTA. Sodium benzoate can form small amounts of benzene, a known carcinogen, when combined with vitamin C under heat and light, and this has triggered recalls in the past. Potassium sorbate helps suppress mold and yeast but can cause headaches, rashes, and stomach upset in sensitive people. EDTA acts as a chelator, tying up metals and stabilizing color, but it can also interfere with the body's own mineral balance and sometimes aggravate digestion.

Cheaper teas, herbal blends, and bottled energy drinks from lower income countries often enter global markets with little independent testing. Each year, authorities recall imported beverages for banned pesticides, excessive heavy metals, or unapproved plant ingredients, and some detox teas and energy shots have caused poisoning, liver injury, or psychiatric symptoms because they contained potent unlisted herbs or drugs. No agency has the capacity to test every shipment of every drink, which means many products reach shelves essentially unexamined.

Sugar and sweeteners are layered on top of all this. A single sixteen ounce bottle of iced tea or soda typically contains around 40 grams of sugar or more, exceeding the daily added sugar limit many health agencies recommend. Ready to drink coffees, cold brews, and energy teas often add high fructose corn syrup, sucralose, aspartame, or acesulfame potassium; high sugar intake is tightly tied to obesity, diabetes, fatty liver, and heart disease, while long term data on artificial sweeteners link them to cardiovascular risk, disrupted gut bacteria, and higher rates of weight gain and metabolic syndrome despite their low calories. Large doses of caffeine plus sugar in children and teens raise blood pressure and stress hormones and have been associated with hospitalizations for heart rhythm problems, seizures, and acute mental health crises after energy drink binges.

Chronic exposure to heavy metals and mycotoxins in tea and coffee can quietly damage health over years. Studies have found that many brewed teas provide enough lead to exceed recommended limits in pregnancy if consumed daily, and early life exposure to cadmium, arsenic, and mercury has been linked to higher risks of developmental issues, learning problems, autoimmune disease, and some cancers. Mycotoxins often go unnoticed in taste but may contribute to headaches, fatigue, mood changes, and flares of allergy or skin problems, particularly in children, people with asthma, and those using very cheap beans from humid regions.

Short term, many drinks contribute to headaches, insomnia, jitters, rapid heartbeat, stomach upset, and cravings. Long term, regular consumption of ultra processed, heavily sweetened and flavored drinks raises the likelihood of diabetes, obesity, hypertension, kidney strain, cognitive decline, hormone imbalance, and a host of medical "mystery" symptoms that are hard to trace back to a single ingredient because they arise from a cocktail of dozens of chemicals, metals, and additives combined in the body over time. That cocktail effect is real and extremely difficult for science to fully measure, because no study can test all the combinations people actually drink in real life.

Ultra processed beverages are marketed as wellness boosters, energy aides, focus enhancers, or calming tonics, but they often hide sedatives, stimulants, psychoactive herbs, or flavor chemicals that have never been thoroughly tested in humans, and some would not be legal if labeled accurately. Children, teens, pregnant women, older adults, and people with heart, metabolic, or immune problems face the highest risks because their systems are more sensitive or already stressed, so exposures that a healthy adult might tolerate for a while can trigger serious problems.

For real health, the safest baseline is filtered or tested spring water. If you drink coffee or tea, it helps to choose products from reputable, single origin growers that publish independent lab tests for metals, molds, and pesticides, and to prepare them at home in glass, ceramic, or stainless steel instead of plastic. Never microwave or heat drinks in plastic containers or bottles, and avoid or strictly limit bottled energy and wellness drinks, especially anything with proprietary blends or ingredient lists you cannot easily understand. Bargain, untraceable, or anonymous imported drinks may look like a deal, but they can cost far more in long term health than they save at the checkout.

The human body now faces beverage risks that did not exist even a few generations ago. From contaminated soil and factory solvents to plastic leaching, unlisted herbs, and heavy metal residues, every sip is part of an ongoing experiment. Once you understand how modern drinks are made, choosing simpler options becomes less about fear and more about self protection, because in the world of today's beverages, ignorance is not bliss; it is a gamble with your health.

Chapter Fifteen

Spices, Condiments, and "Hidden Ingredients" (covers MSG, dyes, emulsifiers, flavorings, salad dressings, and sauce mixes)

Many readers have seen some of these chemical dangers before, but condiments and spice mixes are in a league of their own. These products stack one sneaky ingredient on top of another until the list is longer than a tax form. Most people grab a bottle of ranch or a taco mix thinking it just adds flavor; in reality, each squirt or sprinkle unleashes a parade of additives. If one chemical worries you, wait until you see the full cast hiding behind "sauce" and "seasoning."

MSG is the world's most common flavor bomb and it wears a thousand disguises. Words like autolyzed yeast, hydrolyzed protein, yeast extract, natural flavors, and umami extract often signal added glutamates even when MSG is not listed outright. MSG and related boosters make bland food taste intense, but reports have linked them in some people to headaches, flushing, rapid heartbeat, and tingling sensations, sometimes called Chinese Restaurant Syndrome, while animal work has connected high glutamate intake to obesity, hormone changes, and altered gut brain signaling.

These flavor boosters show up in far more than obvious Asian sauces or chips. Baby foods, frozen dinners, broth cubes, flavored rice packets, cheese puffs, and even some all natural burgers and veggie patties rely on glutamate rich ingredients to keep flavors strong. For some, they drive food cravings and override fullness signals, tricking the brain into wanting more. Experts still debate how often they cause clear symptoms, but analyses continue to find added glutamates in dozens of processed meals and snacks across the grocery store.

If the color of your mustard, hot sauce, or taco sauce looks unnaturally bright, it may not be from peppers or turmeric alone. Synthetic dyes such as Red 40, Yellow 5, Yellow 6, and Blue 1 appear widely in condiments, salad dressings, relishes, pickles, jarred jalapeños, and seasoning packets, and titanium dioxide is used to make white, creamy sauces and ranch dressings look perfectly opaque. European regulators require warnings or limits on several of these dyes because of evidence that some mixtures can worsen hyperactive behavior in susceptible children, and titanium dioxide has been restricted from foods in the European Union over concerns about possible DNA damage.

Keeping sauces creamy and stable is an industrial art. Emulsifiers and stabilizers such as polysorbate 60 or 80, soy lecithin, guar gum, xanthan gum, methylcellulose, and cellulose gum help oil and water stay mixed, keep dressings smooth, and prevent separation. Experimental and animal studies suggest that some commonly used emulsifiers can disturb gut bacteria, thin the protective mucus layer, and promote low grade inflammation, changes that may aggravate weight gain, food sensitivities, and bowel symptoms in people prone to IBS or inflammatory gut disease.

Preservatives are the label anti heroes. Sodium benzoate, potassium sorbate, EDTA, and BHA or BHT show up on many dressing, sauce, and condiment shelves to keep products safe at room temperature. Sodium benzoate can react with vitamin C under heat and light to form small amounts of benzene, a known carcinogen, which has triggered beverage and sauce recalls in the past; potassium sorbate and benzoates can provoke headaches, hives, or asthma like symptoms in some sensitive people. EDTA binds metals and stabilizes color but may also bind minerals in the gut, while BHA and BHT are synthetic antioxidants that some agencies classify as possible carcinogens based on long term animal studies.

Spice packets and cheap rubs carry their own tricks. Anti caking agents such as silicon dioxide and calcium silicate are added to keep powders flowing, and maltodextrin, a refined starch, bulks up blends while spiking their glycemic impact. Investigations have uncovered imported spices adulterated with non food fillers, including ground nutshells or even brick dust, and in some cities, contaminated turmeric and chili powders have caused clusters of lead poisoning in children.

Sugar, salt, and industrial fats hide in most sauces and seasoning kits. High fructose corn syrup or similar syrups sweeten many ketchups, barbecue sauces, and "honey" mustards, and a tablespoon or two can rival a cookie in sugar content. Ranch powder, honey mustard packets, and taco or fajita seasoning mixes often include added sugar, maltodextrin, or stealth sweeteners like stevia or monk fruit, which can be harsh on digestion for some people when combined with gums and fibers.

Organic and natural claims do not automatically make condiments safe. Natural flavors is a legally vague term that can describe concentrates from almost any once living source, including microbes, plants, or animal secretions, modified heavily in labs before ending up in an "authentic" hot sauce or "artisan" dressing. Smoke flavor, essence, and aroma on labels usually mean engineered flavor chemicals, not simple spices or real smoking. Allergies and intolerance to complex flavor mixtures are hard to track because testing on these proprietary blends is rarely done.

Global spice trade adds another layer. Investigations have repeatedly found turmeric, chili powders, and curry mixes tainted with lead chromate, illegal Sudan dyes, or other banned colorants, especially in low cost imports, and baby food and rice products have been recalled after similar contamination. Counterfeit saffron and paprika have been found with textile dyes and non food particles, and when one importer is shut down, the same product may reappear in new packaging under a new brand name.

Label rules help hide this complexity. Words like maltodextrin, spices, seasoning, color, and natural flavors act as umbrella terms that can contain many sub ingredients without being individually named. This allows a jar of salsa or a bottle of sauce to claim no artificial flavors or no artificial colors while still containing multiple highly processed components derived in labs. In general, the longer and more vague the ingredient list, the less you can trust that it reflects a traditional recipe.

Emulsifiers and stabilizers deserve special attention. Polysorbate 80, carrageenan, and cellulose gums have all been studied for their effects on intestinal lining and microbes; some animal models show carrageenan can cause colitis like inflammation and tumor promotion, and emulsifier mixtures have altered microbiota in ways that promote metabolic syndrome and gut inflammation. People with IBS, Crohn's disease, or ulcerative colitis often report worse symptoms when eating heavily emulsified foods, but even people without diagnoses may notice bloating, gas, and fatigue after regular use.

Next time you say just a little ketchup or just a drizzle of dressing, remember that many commercial brands carry more sugar and sodium per tablespoon than you might expect, plus dyes, gums, and preservatives in every squeeze. Ranch seasoning and dip mixes combine MSG type flavor boosters, dairy powders, sugars, starches, and gums; low fat dressings often trade fat for sugar, thickeners, and fibers that do not necessarily improve health. A basic taco seasoning packet can easily list twenty or more ingredients, making one of the simplest home dishes one of the most chemically complex items in the cart.

Science is starting to catch up with what clinicians have suspected. Diets heavy in ultra processed sauces, seasonings, and condiments are associated with higher rates of allergies, hyperactivity in some children, anxiety, metabolic syndrome, hypertension, and autoimmune flares, and emulsifiers and certain dyes are now recognized as likely contributors to gut and behavior problems in susceptible people. Children are especially vulnerable to synthetic colors, preservatives, and emulsifiers because of their smaller bodies and developing brains and immune systems.

Staying safer means learning to decode labels and simplify. If a bottle or packet lists more than a handful of ingredients and most of them are not recognizable foods, putting it back is often wise. Making spice blends from whole seeds and simple dried herbs avoids anti caking agents and hidden fillers, and homemade ranch or vinaigrette with real yogurt or olive oil, lemon, salt, and herbs can be prepared in minutes without gums, dyes, or MSG. Taco night really only needs cumin, paprika or chili, garlic, onion, and salt, not maltodextrin, spice extractives, and flow agents.

A practical tip is to read condiment labels out loud; if you sound like you are reciting a chemistry experiment, you probably are. Choosing clean brands with short, clear ingredient lists or assembling your own dressings and rubs in a jar shifts power back from factories to your kitchen. Seasonings, sauces, and condiments can absolutely enhance food, but they should be based on real ingredients, not a cocktail of unpronounceable compounds. For better health, fewer ingredients, less added color, and more home cooking remain the best seasoning you will find.

Chapter Sixteen

Supplements and Health Foods (powders, bars, deceptive claims, artificial nutrients, fortification, protein isolates)

SUPPLEMENTS AND HEALTH FOODS dominate store shelves, promising everything from quick muscles to sharp brains and healthy hearts. Powders, bars, and gummies fill baskets with bright branding and claims about energy, focus, and wellness, but read the label and you often find an ingredient list that belongs in a lab notebook, not a kitchen. Real dangers hide behind these promises, and pulling back the curtain shows how complex and underregulated this world really is.

FDA and medical researchers keep finding that miracle supplements are not always what they claim. In recent years, hundreds of supplements have been recalled for containing banned drugs, hidden prescription medications, or undeclared allergens, including weight loss pills spiked with stimulants and muscle products laced with steroids. Protein powders, especially plant based blends, are notorious for contamination. Independent testing by groups such as the Clean Label Project has found that a large majority of popular powders contained measurable lead, cadmium, arsenic, or mercury, with plant proteins like pea and rice often testing substantially higher than whey because plants take up more metals from soil. Lead accumulates in the brain, kidneys, and bones and is linked even at low levels to nerve disease, cancer, developmental delay, and memory problems, especially in children and pregnant women.

It gets worse. Some protein powders also test positive for BPA or related plastic chemicals that can leach from tubs, scoops, or processing equipment, raising concerns about hormone disruption, fertility issues, and cancer risk. Independent labs have reported that a significant fraction of plant based powders exceeded California's Prop 65 limits for heavy metals, and a few servings contained several times the safe daily level for lead or arsenic. Yet many people drink these shakes daily at breakfast or after workouts, unaware that each scoop might add to their long term toxic burden.

Bars sit under a health halo but bring industrial baggage. Many high protein or whole food bars are packed with sugar alcohols, gums, processed protein isolates, and fillers. Labels may boast 15 to 20 grams of protein, but that protein often comes with high sodium and low digestibility, while sweeteners such as maltitol, sucralose, or erythritol commonly cause cramping, diarrhea, or bloating in real world use. Recalls have pulled bars from shelves for Salmonella contamination, undeclared nuts or sesame, and hidden drugs, and energy or "pre workout" bars with added caffeine and herbs have sent teens and young adults to the emergency room with liver injury, heart palpitations, or arrhythmias.

Artificial fibers, cheap thickeners, processed gums, and palm oil are major filler risks. Inulin, polydextrose, and similar added fibers can create an illusion of high fiber while provoking gas, pain, and diarrhea for many people, especially those with sensitive guts. Palm oil and hydrogenated or heavily refined fats extend shelf life and improve texture, but they often raise LDL cholesterol and can promote inflammation when they displace healthier fats and whole foods, raising the risk over time for high blood pressure, heart disease, and stroke. Many bars and powders also rely on generic vegetable oils, typically soybean or canola, which in ultra processed form are associated with markers of metabolic stress when consumed in large amounts as part of a Western diet.

Fortified foods and supplements load store aisles with synthetic vitamins and minerals, but more is not always better. High dose vitamin B6 supplements have been linked to nerve damage, numbness, and burning or tingling sensations in long term users, and too much vitamin A or iron in people who are not deficient can contribute to bone problems, headaches, and liver injury. Daily use of multiple fortified bars, drinks, and pills can quietly push intakes of certain B vitamins or fat soluble vitamins into ranges associated with insomnia, anxiety, rapid heart rate, or other side effects.

Label loopholes make all of this harder to see. Phrases like proprietary blend, matrix, or complex mean you do not know the actual amount of each ingredient; brands can sprinkle tiny, ineffective doses of trendy botanicals such as ashwagandha, acai, or goji while highlighting them on the front of the package. Natural flavors and doctor recommended banners remind you how little premarket testing is required for most supplements under U.S. law; the FDA generally steps in only after people are harmed. Manufacturers can change suppliers or tweak formulas between batches with minimal oversight, and many products are never tested by independent labs.

Recalls are soaring and safety is not guaranteed, even from well known brands. Recent warning letters and enforcement actions have covered products tainted with Listeria, undeclared peanuts or sesame, banned stimulants, and unapproved drugs, including some marketed for energy, cognitive enhancement, or rapid weight loss. Pediatric poison centers report serious incidents from iron rich gummies and chewables when children accidentally eat too many, sometimes requiring hospital care and antidotes. High energy or fat burning supplements have been implicated in cases of heart attacks, strokes, seizures, and sudden death in young, otherwise healthy adults.

Synthetic sweeteners such as sucralose, aspartame, and acesulfame potassium often sneak into bars and powders to keep calories low while preserving intense sweetness. Large cohort and mechanistic studies link high intakes of artificial sweeteners and diet drinks with increased risk of cardiovascular disease, metabolic syndrome, and changes to gut microbiota, and many users report headaches, digestive upset, or mood changes. Gums and fake fibers like inulin or resistant dextrins may worsen IBS symptoms, causing cramping, gas, and bloating, and long term exposure to heavy additive loads appears to alter gut bacteria in ways that may drive inflammation and new food intolerances for some people.

The all natural or organic illusion often crumbles under independent testing. Analyses of organic plant based blends have found pesticide residues in a sizable fraction of products, and so called superfood greens frequently turn out to be powdered spinach, pea hulls, and grasses mixed with natural colorants and a long list of stabilizers and flavors. Organic labeling rules allow a certain percentage of non organic ingredients in multi component products, so an "organic" powder can still contain synthetic fillers, conventional flavors, and additives alongside its organic components.

Sodium levels in meal bars and drinks can easily hit 300 to 400 milligrams per serving, pushing blood pressure up in salt sensitive individuals and adding to kidney strain. Fats listed simply as healthy blend or vegetable oil may include palm kernel oil, refined canola, or small amounts of residual trans fats; months of regular use can worsen cholesterol ratios and subtly increase appetite, undermining weight control goals.

Major health organizations now warn that some protein supplements and so called health foods are among the leading hidden sources of heavy metal exposure in younger adults, and chronic low level lead and arsenic intake is tied to brain fog, kidney problems, bone pain, and increased cardiovascular risk. Very high intakes of vitamin D or B12 from overlapping products can trigger rashes, headaches, elevated blood pressure, and in rare cases more serious neurologic symptoms.

Even with warnings and recurring scandals, sales keep climbing. Fat burning supplements have repeatedly been found to contain unlisted amphetamine like compounds or other stimulants, and emergency physicians view them as a significant risk factor for sudden cardiovascular events in young adults who mix them with exercise, caffeine, or dehydration. People who must avoid gluten, dairy, soy, or eggs are often drawn to free from claims on bars and powders, but the replacements typically include dozens of new chemicals, gums, flavors, and sweetener mixes, each with its own potential for side effects and cross reactions.

Many users of protein powders and health bars eventually report headaches, constipation, anxiety, insomnia, swelling, chest tightness, or inexplicable fatigue. When they stop or sharply reduce highly processed supplements and shift toward whole foods, many notice rapid improvements in digestion, energy, and even skin and joint symptoms, because the body recognizes nutrients from real food and can regulate vitamin and mineral uptake better when they arrive in an apple or a handful of almonds instead of a fortified shake.

The safest recipe to avoid the worst outcomes is simple. Base your diet on real, minimally processed foods, and treat bars and powders as occasional tools for genuine medical needs or true athletic demands, not as everyday meal replacements. If you do choose supplements, look for third party seals such as USP, NSF, or Informed Choice, which indicate independent testing for purity, label accuracy, and banned substances.

Be wary of labels that boast proprietary blend, matrix, pro complex, raw, or doctor formulated without disclosing exact amounts, and skip anything sold as miracle, extreme, or quick fix. Products with short ingredient lists full of recognizable foods are generally safer bets. Remember that some of the most dramatic ER stories and recall headlines began with someone just following directions on a flashy label. You do not need superhero shakes or bioengineered blends; for most people, real food, clean water, movement, and time are still the real secret sauce for lasting health.

Chapter Seventeen

Baby Food, Infant Formula, Snacks, and Sippy-Cup Surprises

WALK THE BABY FOOD aisle and you see jars, pouches, and formula tubs lined up in cheery rows, each one promising to help your little one grow. It looks safe and specially made for infants, but beneath the bright packaging are real shocks: heavy metals, hidden sugars, synthetic nutrients, plastics, and factory germs. Most baby foods and formulas are made in large plants, cooked at high heat, dried, blended, and processed until little remains of the original fruit, vegetable, or grain, while snack puffs, yogurt melts, teething rice, and squeeze pouches often deliver more added sugar, starches, and thickeners than genuine nutrition.

Scientists keep finding heavy metals such as lead, arsenic, mercury, and cadmium in baby food and formula. A widely cited Congressional investigation reported some products with lead dozens of times higher than bottled water limits and arsenic and cadmium far above recommended levels, and independent tests have found that the vast majority of sampled baby foods contained at least one metal. These contaminants show up in infant rice cereal, formula, pouches, snacks, and cereals from familiar brands, and early life exposure to heavy metals is associated with lower IQ, ADHD, learning difficulties, and higher risks for long term brain and behavior issues.

The sources are everywhere: polluted soil, old water pipes, contaminated machinery, and the crops themselves. Arsenic tends to accumulate in rice, which is why infant rice cereal has been heavily criticized, while lead can contaminate fruit and vegetable mixtures through irrigation water and residues in processing plants. Fast growing baby food categories such as squeeze pouches and powdered “on the go” snacks can deliver levels of sugar and metals that would trigger concern in adult foods, yet are often marketed as gentle and convenient.

Plastics, hormones, and so called forever chemicals hide in the packaging and tools used around baby food. BPA, phthalates, and microplastics have been detected in formula powders, can linings, bottle nipples, and pouches, and preparing hot formula in polypropylene bottles can release large numbers of microplastic particles into a single feeding. These chemicals are linked to hormonal disruption, reduced fertility, immune changes, and higher cancer risk, and because babies have small bodies and rapidly developing organs, they can receive months’ worth of exposure in a short time from repeated feedings.

Bacteria and mold are another quiet threat. Recent high profile recalls of powdered formulas followed detection of dangerous organisms such as Cronobacter and, in rare cases, Clostridium species in powdered products, with some infants developing severe infections, meningitis, or dying after consumption. Even minor failures in factory sanitation, cracks in pipes, or poor hand hygiene can contaminate an entire batch, and powdered formula is not sterile, so unsafe handling or storage at home can add further risk.

Big name and store brand baby foods commonly use synthetic vitamins and fortifiers. Lab made iron, DHA for brain and eye claims, B12, and other added nutrients are mixed in so companies can advertise brain boost or immune support. Babies do not always absorb these forms well, and some formulas also contain thickeners such as guar gum, carrageenan, and modified starches that can bloat small tummies or worsen reflux and constipation. Toddler snacks and flavored pouches may also contain artificial colors, preservatives, or intense sweeteners disguised under natural flavor and fruit concentrate wording.

On the shelf, nearly every jar and pouch seems reassuring, labeled all natural, non GMO, organic, or doctor recommended, but labels do not have to list heavy metals or microplastics, and many companies do not routinely test for them. Products recalled or restricted in other countries may still be sold in U.S. stores, and claims like contains DHA or supports brain development are often allowed without strong proof they improve real world outcomes. Marketing language can easily outpace science and regulation.

Snacking has become step two for many babies. Puffs, mini crackers, yogurt melts, and toddler cookies are typically made from refined rice or corn, added sugar, natural flavors, and processed thickeners, and analyses show some of these snacks contain more heavy metals per gram than typical adult foods. Baby juices and toddler drinks often carry more sugar and acid than soda, setting children up for future diabetes, heart risk, and cavities, while teaching the palate to prefer bland, oversweet, ultra processed foods instead of real textures and flavors.

Real families' experiences make the data tangible. Parents have reported developmental delays, mood changes, or regression after months on certain jarred foods or snacks, and lawsuits have pushed companies and regulators toward transparency. States like California are implementing rules that will require clearer heavy metal information by mid decade, and federal agencies are slowly tightening limits and guidance, but progress is uneven and often lags behind emerging evidence.

Parents can reduce risk by making targeted swaps. Simple homemade baby food steamed and mashed vegetables or fruits avoids many contaminants and additives, especially when made from diverse ingredients rather than relying heavily on rice. When preparing formula, using cool, filtered water and glass bottles when possible can lower exposure to metals and plastic particles. Minimizing "just add water" snacks and squeeze pouches, avoiding added sugar in first foods, and choosing packaged products with very short ingredient lists, without rice, added sugar, flavors, colors, or thickeners high on the label, all help.

No snack or pouch should be a child's main first food. Buying frozen whole vegetables and fruits, cooking them at home, and freezing small portions in ice cube trays can provide convenient, safer options. Asking a pediatrician which vitamins truly matter and being cautious about hype around single magic ingredients is important, as is favoring quality glass jars or thoroughly vetted brands over convenience plastics when possible. Local or small brands that publish third party testing and transparent results give more accountability than anonymous mass products.

Checking safety recalls regularly through official or consumer sites helps parents respond quickly if a product is flagged. If a baby develops unexplained rash, constipation, poor appetite, sleep changes, or behavior shifts, food and formula should be on the list of things to review with a pediatrician. Sharing concerns with other parents and caregivers raises awareness and pressure for safer products. Above all, marketing should not override common sense: babies' first foods are best when they are simple, whole, and low in sugar, sodium, and chemicals, because those early bites can shape health for years.

Chapter Eighteen

Pet Food and Household Items: Hidden risks from pet foods, cleaners, and non-food items sold in groceries

THE STORY OF PET food is not just about what animals should not eat, but how a booming industry has turned feeding them into a science experiment and a shopping event. The push to avoid "people food" often keeps owners returning for premium, scientifically formulated, or ancestral kibbles and canned diets, while the United States now counts tens of millions of dogs and cats and spends tens of billions of dollars each year on pet food alone.

Many forbidden foods for pets are real dangers: chocolate, onions, garlic, grapes and raisins, macadamia nuts, raw dough, and xylitol sweetened treats can cause everything from vomiting and seizures to organ failure and emergency vet visits. Yet just a generation ago, many household pets lived on table scraps and simple leftovers, while today owners are more likely to purchase single protein, grain free, or limited ingredient diets, subscribe to delivery boxes, and buy pet insurance. Pet hospital visits have shifted from parasites and trauma to chronic issues such as allergies, itchy skin, long term digestive upset, diabetes, and suspected food intolerances, often managed with specialty diets, prescription treats, and supplements.

A look inside modern pet food reveals highly processed recipes. Typical dry foods feature meat by products or meat meals rendered at high heat, fish meal, beef tallow, ground corn, corn gluten meal, soy protein isolates, and flavor sprays, plus multiple preservatives like BHA, propyl gallate, menadione, citric acid, and tocopherols. Artificial colors and whitening agents such as caramel color, Red 40, and titanium dioxide are used to make kibbles and gravies visually appealing to humans. Independent testing has found concerning levels of heavy metals in some top selling brands, including lead, arsenic, and mercury, often from fish and grain byproducts, while past scandals with melamine adulterated wheat gluten and aflatoxin contaminated corn have caused large recalls and thousands of pet deaths.

Packaging adds further risks. Cans, trays, and flexible pouches can contain BPA, phthalates, and other chemicals that migrate into fatty foods, potentially disrupting hormones in pets over years of daily feeding. Even BPA free claims do not guarantee safety, because replacement linings can use similar bisphenols with less research behind them. Treats and wet foods packaged in soft plastics sometimes show pesticide residues from imported ingredients and cross contamination on shared factory lines. At the same time, microbiological hazards are common: dry and raw pet foods and treats are frequently recalled for Salmonella, Listeria, or E. coli, causing illness in animals and sometimes in people who handle the products or live in the same home.

Household products stored near pet food can also endanger animals. Bleach, ammonia cleaners, pine oil, citrus based sprays, and essential oil diffusers can poison pets if licked from fur or paws, with cats especially sensitive to many oils. Carpet powders, floor polishes, and odor neutralizing candles can leave residues that irritate the liver and kidneys. Dryer sheets and fabric softeners contain cationic surfactants and fragrances that are toxic if chewed, and cocoa mulch, rodent poisons, and detergent pods that smell interesting or resemble toys have all sent pets to emergency clinics with seizures, chemical burns, or organ failure. Every year, animal poison hotlines handle hundreds of thousands of calls, most for accidental exposure to common household items.

Boutique, imported, and raw style treats can be just as risky as mass market products. Foreign sourced jerky and chews have been recalled for antibiotic residues, undisclosed allergens, toxins, and contamination and have been linked to kidney syndromes and deaths in dogs. Raw and exotic protein diets often test high for bacteria and bone fragments and, in some cases, heavy metals. Grain free kibbles built on peas, lentils, and potatoes were tied to a surge in dilated cardiomyopathy in certain dog breeds, prompting an official investigation into diet related heart disease. Ingredient lists have grown longer as brands add pea protein, legumes, chia, flavor extracts, and "superfoods" to stand out, but many are not subject to robust third party testing or traceable sourcing.

Given all this, owners reasonably ask whether modern risk is worth it when earlier generations of pets lived on simpler fare. As animals have moved from yards to bedrooms and from barn duty to family status, industry product lines have multiplied into probiotic chews, calming biscuits, vitamin powders, superfood kibbles, and freeze dried toppers. What is still often missing is clear, honest information about what goes into each bag and how it is tested.

To keep pets safer, it helps to choose brands that are transparent about ingredients and sourcing, use relatively short labels, provide clear lot numbers, and share independent testing or quality certifications. Avoid bargain and imported snacks with vague origins or no way to contact the maker. Store food and treats away from cleaners, pesticides, and medicines, wash hands after feeding or handling raw or moist foods, and discard products promptly if they smell rancid, appear moldy, or are part of a recall. If you cannot easily find contact details or batch information, or if claims sound too good to be true, it is wise to look elsewhere.

Veterinarians now routinely treat pets for diabetes, chronic vomiting or diarrhea, unexplained allergies, and persistent skin and liver problems, and many owners purchase costly imaging, specialty consults, and insurance just to manage conditions that may be influenced by long term diet. The verdict is that while modern pets often live longer and more pampered lives, they also face new, largely invisible dangers every time a bag is opened or a fancy treat is unwrapped. Careful brand selection, safe storage, hand hygiene, regular veterinary partnership, and a cautious eye toward the latest miracle mix offer the best chance to give four legged family members longer, healthier lives, one bowl at a time.

Chapter Nineteen

Water and Ice (bottled water, microplastics, tap water, PFAS, filtration issues)

IN EARLIER CHAPTERS WE picked apart the dangers of plastic packaging in food, so this chapter on water and ice goes straight to the bottle. When you walk down the grocery aisle, it is almost impossible to find water in glass; plastic rules. Each bottle is missing a real timeline, a chart showing when and how long it has been sitting since it left the ground or a municipal tap. Bottled water has no made on date, no travel log, and the only real guarantee is a long shelf life, sometimes listed as up to two years, all that time leaching chemicals from its container.

Many buyers trust bottled water because it looks pure and is packaged fresh. The truth is far less magic. Nearly two thirds of bottled water in the United States is just treated municipal tap water, run through extra filters, then rebottled and marked up to enormous prices. Some companies boast about artesian or mountain sources yet frequently refill their tanks with the same city water everyone else gets. Labels might add phrases such as enhanced with minerals or triple filtered, but rarely explain that the added minerals often include basic table salt or calcium to make it taste less flat. To top it off, chlorination or fluoride used for safety and taste may still be present, sometimes unlisted.

If you have ever looked at bottled water and wondered about tiny floating bits, you are not alone. Research estimates that people who drink mostly bottled water consume tens of thousands more microplastic particles per year than those who stick to tap. A single liter of bottled water can contain anywhere from a few hundred to hundreds of thousands of plastic fragments, most invisible to the naked eye. Unlike food, water's microplastics come not just from the bottle but from the cap and the bottling machines themselves. The smaller the fragment, the higher the chance it slips through our defenses and finds a home in the bloodstream or organs. Scientists now point to these particles as potential triggers for inflammation, hormone changes, reproductive trouble, cancer, and long term brain or gut injury.

Bottled water is also a playground for invisible chemicals. The FDA regulates bottled water, but EPA rules for tap water are stricter. Tap water is tested frequently, often daily or hundreds of times per month, and cities must publicly report violations and problems. Bottled water companies can test far less often and usually only in large batches, and they are only required to meet certain standards if the product crosses state lines.

Chemical leaching from bottles is real and gets worse over time or with a little heat. Sun in the car, a warm truck, or a hot room in August can raise antimony, bisphenols, and phthalate levels many fold. These substances, linked to hormone disruption, cancer, and gut damage, begin moving into water after just a few months in plastic. If you have ever noticed a musty or sweet plastic taste in old water, that is the flavor of time and chemistry at work.

Shelf life is largely a marketing trick. Water itself does not go bad, but bottles do. After three to six months, bacteria can grow if the bottle has been opened even once. Mold and even drug resistant microbes can form films on bottle walls in just days, especially if bottles are refilled or left warm. Fragments of flavor, literally, may come from bottle scratches or repeated use of the same disposable bottle.

PFAS, or forever chemicals, get their name because they never fully leave the environment or the body. Studies have found PFAS in a large share of U.S. bottled waters, and some brands tested higher than nearby tap. These compounds can interfere with hormones, lower fertility, disrupt thyroid function, and are linked to certain cancers. In some testing, sparkling and flavored waters had more PFAS than plain tap water, especially after storage or when carbonation was added. So much for fresh mountain spring.

Microplastic and PFAS exposure is not just a health story; it is a regulation problem. The EPA and FDA operate under different standards and rules. The EPA requires daily testing and public reporting for city water, with limits on more than 90 contaminants. Bottled water may only be tested weekly or by batch, with no obligation to publish results or explain source changes. Marketing words such as natural or mineral do not guarantee that water is either of those things, and the actual source is often hidden behind a code or a vague phrase.

The water you buy may have started its journey months or years ago, bottled and shipped from several states away or even from overseas. By the time it leaves the shelf, microplastics and leached chemicals have had plenty of time to accumulate. This issue is even worse for big water bottles, the multi gallon jugs used in coolers. Studies show microplastic and chemical concentrations rise after repeated refills and long storage times.

Not all bottled water is the same. Glass bottles, still rare but more popular, usually contain fewer microplastic particles, although caps and seals can still contribute plastic residues. Cardboard packages and so called eco bottles often have thin plastic linings that leach their own flavors and chemicals.

Health risks are not abstract. Scientific reviews connect bottled water microplastics to chronic inflammation, oxidative stress, reproductive changes, and possible neurological effects. Children and pregnant people are especially sensitive; tiny plastic particles and persistent chemicals can cross the placenta into unborn babies. PFAS damage hormone systems with special risks for low birth weight, thyroid problems, cholesterol changes, and immune disruption.

A little bacteria does not scare most people, but bottled water's long shelf life can be a perfect setup for unpleasant microbes. After sitting in a warehouse, store, or car, heat and time can turn a bottle into a small petri dish. Researchers have found potent drug resistant bacteria in used or long stored plastic bottles. Any visible cloudiness, odd scent, or off taste is a good reason to throw a bottle away. Longevity in a sealed bottle is not a virtue by itself; freshness, temperature, and cleanliness matter more.

Tap water is not perfect, but it usually faces more scrutiny. EPA limits and daily testing mean city water is more quickly flagged for E. coli, heavy metals, or other violations, and utilities are required to issue boil notices and fix problems. You can find out where your tap water comes from, how often it is tested, and see detailed yearly reports about contaminants and treatment. Bottled water almost never comes with this kind of transparent record.

Marketing spins every label, promising mountain spring or pure glacier. The reality is that the source is often the same municipal supply that flows from your kitchen sink. Added minerals and extra filtration can change taste, but they do not guarantee removal of every plastic particle, every chemical, or all traces of heavy metals.

How can you protect yourself? Filter your tap water with a certified system designed to reduce lead, PFAS, and other contaminants, including some microplastics. Store water in glass or stainless steel bottles and containers when you can. Keep water cool and away from direct sun and heat, and avoid drinking from bottles left in warm cars or sitting for months. The best option for health and the environment is not more plastic, but smarter choices. Filter and store water safely, know the risks, and read the fine print behind every fresh looking bottle in the aisle.

Regularly rotate any stored water and do not let opened bottles sit for days. Wash reusable bottles daily with hot, soapy water and let them dry completely. In emergencies, bottled water has an important place, but everyday hydration deserves better. Each sip of grocery store water may look clear, but what you cannot see can still harm your body over time. In the market, fresh is only as good as storage, source, and honesty allow. Choose wisely, drink safely, and remember that clear does not always mean clean.

Chapter Twenty

Organic Truths and Grocery Store Myths

Many shoppers now see organic as the gold standard. It is often the safest and least polluted option in the grocery store, yet few people really know what the label means or why it costs more. Buzzwords can be misleading, and the extra price is a mystery for many.

The meaning of organic is not as simple as no chemicals. To carry the USDA Organic seal, at least 95 percent of a product's ingredients must meet federal organic certification rules, which prohibit synthetic pesticides, herbicides, chemical fertilizers, routine hormones, and genetically modified organisms. Items labeled 100 percent organic are stricter and use only organic ingredients. Made with organic goes lower and can include just 70 percent organic content. The remaining 30 percent can include non-organic agricultural ingredients from the USDA's allowed list, such as cornstarch, unbleached lecithin, gums like guar and locust bean, pectin, certain dairy cultures, and some minerals, and these must not be genetically modified, irradiated, or fertilized with sewage sludge.

What about that extra 30 percent? Some of the most common non-organic additives include carrageenan, a thickener from seaweed that some health advocates believe can upset digestion. Other allowed substances, like calcium chloride, are used in canned tomatoes and beans, while citric acid and certain enzymes often show up in bread, cereal, or yogurt. Synthetic ingredients such as ascorbic acid and xanthan gum, though originally derived from natural sources, are processed in factories into commercial products. If a product's organic ingredients fall short or there is a shortage, companies can request waivers to use non-organic versions if they argue that an organic form is not commercially available, and inspectors are supposed to verify this but enforcement can vary across the food chain.

Can these approved non-organic ingredients harm health? It depends on the ingredient and the person. Some, like carrageenan or certain gums, can cause gut upset in sensitive individuals. Research has suggested that some food gums, mineral acids, or synthetic vitamins may contribute to digestive trouble, allergies, or, in rare cases, stronger reactions. The main concern is less about acute poisoning and more about chronic accumulation of processed elements in foods that shoppers assume are simple and pure. For example, flavored organic soy or almond milks can contain many non-organic additives, some of which consumer advocates have flagged as potential concerns for digestion or long-term exposure.

Animal products labeled organic must follow rules about housing, health care, feed, and bans on routine antibiotics and synthetic growth hormones. However, organic livestock feed can include imported grains such as soybeans or corn. Investigations have found that a large share of organic soy used for feed in the United States is imported, which opens the door to fraud, mislabeling, or hidden genetically modified feed that never appears on consumer labels.

Packaging adds another layer. An organic item can be packed, and still stay certified, in plastic, lined cans, or cartons with chemical coatings. Organic rules focus on how food is grown and processed, not on packaging materials or the migration of chemicals from that packaging into the food. That means organic beans, berries, or juices may still pick up BPA, phthalates, or microplastics during processing, shipping, and storage.

Processed organic foods can also use up to five percent non-organic content. This portion typically includes items that are difficult to find in organic form, such as baking soda, citric acid, ascorbic acid, certain stabilizers, or cultures. They must still meet core criteria—no genetic engineering, no irradiation, no sewage sludge—but during supply shortages or with waivers, conventional versions may be used. Consumer watchdogs have noted that enforcement often weakens when demand surges and companies argue an organic version is unavailable.

Labeling sounds strong, but the reality in stores is more complicated. Products with the USDA Organic seal can still contain up to five percent non-organic ingredients, which can include gelling agents, colors, and flavors never grown on organic farms. Made with organic on the front panel allows up to 30 percent non-organic content as long as the seal is not used and those ingredients appear on the allowed list. Many imported products call themselves organic, but inspections may be infrequent, and paperwork errors, fraud, or relabeling are documented problems, especially in big export categories like coffee, nuts, grains, and honey.

Food fraud is booming. In one of the United States' largest organic fraud cases, a Missouri grain dealer sold hundreds of millions of dollars' worth of conventional crops as organic before going to prison. Other schemes in Midwestern states added tens of millions more in fake organic grain to the market. Globally, reports indicate that food fraud has grown sharply in recent years, with organic mislabeling a recurring theme, driven by high demand, limited true supply, and the price premium consumers are willing to pay.

Government checks have shown how porous the system can be. In one survey, nearly half of tested organic produce samples contained pesticide residues not allowed under the organic program. Some contamination came from wind drift or shared equipment, but in other cases, suppliers appear to have relabeled conventional goods to earn higher prices. Major brands and retailers have faced lawsuits, recalls, or fines for misuse of the label, and the USDA regularly posts cases of suspended or revoked organic certificates and counterfeit paperwork.

Even within the rules, organic does not mean chemical free. Exceptions allow certain waxes, cleaning agents, enzymes, and preservatives in broths, juices, and canned items. Organic juice may come from certified oranges but still be pasteurized, stored for months in tanks, and blended with flavor packs or essential oil fractions to keep taste consistent year-round. Organic canned beans may contain added salt, calcium chloride, or a non-organic thickener. Frozen organic strawberries can travel across the globe in plastic and retain certification as long as the originating farm and processor are certified.

Natural on a label, by contrast, has almost no regulatory meaning. It typically means only that the product does not contain artificial flavors or colors, and it offers no protection from pesticides, growth hormones, or industrial farming practices. Cage free eggs often come from birds housed indoors without cages but still in crowded barns, and grass fed beef might spend only part of its life on pasture before confinement feeding. Claims like humanely raised and free range can vary widely in practice and are often loosely defined.

Price is the shopper's warning sign. On average, organic fruits and vegetables cost around half again as much as conventional, eggs can cost substantially more, and meat, milk, and bread often run from 20 to 100 percent higher. Organic farming usually requires more labor, crop rotation, manual weed control, and costly certification, and yields can drop during the years it takes to transition from conventional. Fees for inspections and compliance can reach hundreds or thousands of dollars per year, and combined with weather and pest risks, this can squeeze small farmers and limit supply.

But the price difference is not always just about cost. High demand, limited supplies, and consumer willingness to pay premiums also raise prices. Imports fill many U.S. supermarket organic shelves, but enforcement gaps mean that lower-quality or questionably produced goods from abroad can appear under U.S. organic labels. When a large fraction of organic feed, such as soybeans, is imported, tracing authenticity becomes harder and opportunities for fraud expand. Shipments may move primarily on paper, with physical checks catching only a fraction of mislabeling.

So why choose organic at all? Long-term studies and meta--analyses show that, on average, organic produce and milk have lower pesticide residues, less frequent contamination with antibiotic-resistant bacteria, and reduced exposure to some synthetic additives and antibiotics. Organic management can improve soil quality, reduce some environmental pollutants, and support pollinators and biodiversity better than many conventional systems. Animal welfare standards tend to be higher than in standard industrial operations. Surveys show that a large majority of shoppers view organic as the most meaningful front-of-pack claim, even though many do not fully understand the exact standard.

For personal health, organic is usually the safer bet, but label literacy still matters. Fresh, single-ingredient organic foods—fruits, vegetables, whole grains, eggs, and nuts offer the clearest benefits and the fewest label loopholes. Bulk bins, heavily processed organic cookies, energy bars, or meat substitutes can still contain a significant proportion of non-organic or highly processed components. When shopping, looking for the USDA Organic seal, noting the certifying agency, and checking country of origin all help. Supporting local, direct-from-farm sources or trusted co-ops reduces the distance and number of middlemen where cheating can occur. Deeply discounted "organic" imports at big box stores deserve extra scrutiny.

The organic aisle offers both real protection and occasional misdirection. You cannot fix every flaw in the system, but staying aware, reading labels, and asking questions help you get more of the value you are paying for. Organic remains the safest mainstream label for limiting invisible farm chemicals, but knowledge is still your best defense. In a world full of marketing claims, wisdom in the produce and packaged-food aisles pays off every time you shop.

Chapter Twenty-One

The Great Farmers Market Deception: Trust, Verify, and Protect Your Wallet

THE FARMERS' MARKET HAS become a modern American ritual. Saturday mornings, people grab coffee, reusable bags, and a sense of virtue. They walk past colorful tents believing they are buying food straight from the hands that grew it. The story is compelling and straightforward: local farmers, sustainable practices, chemical free produce, handcrafted goods, and prices higher than supermarket prices but "worth it" because they support small farms and healthier food.

That story sells incredibly well. Customers may pay two to three times supermarket prices because they are not just buying tomatoes or honey; they are buying a feeling: freshness, safety, authenticity, and a clean conscience. Very few stop to ask hard questions because the storylines align perfectly with what they want to believe about where their food comes from.

The reality, however, is far uglier. Across the country, investigations by journalists, state agencies, and consumer advocates have documented systematic fraud at farmers' markets. This is not just a handful of bad actors. In many markets, a significant share of vendors are not farmers; they are middlemen operating elaborate repackaging operations. They buy seconds and surplus from wholesale distributors before dawn, rip off the labels, and resell the product as "fresh from our farm."

What looks like a direct connection between you and a local farmer is, all too often, just another supply chain with more lies and a nicer story. Take Cleveland's West Side Market or similar city markets as working examples. From the customer side of the table, it looks wholesome: crates of peppers, beautiful berries, shiny eggplants, and the vendor in a ball cap talking about "the farm." On the vendor side, the day starts very differently.

Long before sunrise, while most shoppers are still asleep, many of these "farmers" are at the wholesale docks. They are not harvesting; they are shopping. Many buy what the grocery chains do not want: seconds and surplus, the boxes that must sell right away or rot because the produce did not meet the size, appearance, or timing needs of big retailers. As a result, vendors purchase it at about half the regular retail price.

By the time you see it, that same produce has been stacked into charming wooden crates, with maybe a chalkboard sign that reads "Fresh This Morning." It looks that way. The problem is that seconds only look good for a very short time. They are already past their shelf life when they arrive at the dock. Chemical treatments used during growing and post harvest handling can help them maintain appearance during trucking and storage, but they cannot stop the clock.

You can see the truth in your own refrigerator. Those gorgeous "just picked" strawberries you brought home on Saturday? By Tuesday, they are collapsing into mush. Cucumbers, squash, and peppers that were "picked yesterday" start to wrinkle, mold, or rot in just a few days. When you grow these crops yourself and refrigerate them, they often last one to two weeks easily. The difference is freshness and honesty.

There are other visual clues right in front of you. Look past the tomatoes and look at the person selling them. Does the "farmer" look like someone who spends dawn to dusk working fields, or like someone who just stepped out of a corner store? Is he leaning against the back of an SUV, sneaking a cigarette behind the tent, surrounded by pristine cardboard boxes? Does he look like the same guy you might see running an inner city convenience store that sells lottery tickets, beer, chips, sugary drinks, and single cigarettes out of a pack?

There is nothing wrong with any of those jobs. But that is not what a full time vegetable farmer's life looks like. Your farmer should look and act like a farmer: weathered, specific, knowledgeable, and just a little too busy to stand around posing as one. To support their performance, many vendors maintain what are better termed "display gardens." Maybe it is a small plot behind their house, or a neatly arranged hoop house with a few rows of tomatoes and herbs. It photographs beautifully. Those photos end up everywhere: on business cards, on social media, and in booth announcements. To the casual eye, it looks like real production.

A typical busy vendor moves 300 to 500 pounds of produce every week. Many attend multiple markets on Friday, Saturday, Sunday, and sometimes more in peak season. A thousand square foot backyard garden cannot come close to feeding that machine. To sustain those volumes week after week, you need acres under cultivation, irrigation, equipment, crop rotation plans, and serious labor. What you see in the glossy photos is a prop. The real source of inventory is somewhere else entirely.

That "somewhere else" is often an Amish or regional produce auction. Scattered across Ohio, Pennsylvania, and neighboring states, these auctions function as centralized wholesale hubs. Amish and other farmers bring truckloads of produce, often from large, highly productive fields. Buyers, including many "farmers' market vendors," show up, bid, and haul away pallet after pallet in the same waxed, labeled boxes you would find in the back of a supermarket.

The economics are irresistible. Bulk lots are priced at wholesale, well below market rates. Vendors load their trucks with these boxes, drive straight to town, strip off the labels, and begin the transformation. Out go the branded cartons. In come weathered looking wooden crates and baskets, maybe a little straw tucked around the edges for effect. The same tomatoes that looked like warehouse inventory an hour ago are now "from our family farm." Sometimes you can find the truth by watching the parking lot rather than the tent. Peek into the back of the truck: are there stacks of identical cardboard boxes with barcodes and brand names? Are workers transferring produce from those boxes into the charming baskets you see out front? The story on the sign and the one on the stone in the truck bed are often different.

And if you are wondering, "Why don't the Amish just come and sell directly?" the answer is that some do, but often not in the way customers imagine. An Amish farmer might have twenty acres of nothing but garlic, or a massive field of onions. They are specialists. Their business model is moving large volumes of one or two crops, not hauling small mixed loads of twenty varieties every weekend. They sell wholesale because they have too much of one item and not enough variety to fill a market stand that resembles a supermarket produce section. So the real farmers stay at the auctions, and the middlemen take it from there.

Produce is only the beginning. Honey fraud is one of the most profitable scams at farmers' markets. The script is simple: buy cheap imported honey in bulk, often cut with rice syrup or corn syrup. The product is rebottled in attractive glass jars labeled "Local Wildflower Honey" or "State Name Apiaries." Real, single source, local honey costs about three times as much at wholesale as this adulterated blend. That price gap is a pure incentive to cheat.

The labels are crafted to evoke emotion: hand drawn bees, barns, wildflowers, and perhaps a family name. The product inside the jar may never have been exposed to a local flower, let alone a local hive. Lab tests and news investigations have often found that a large share of "local" market honey fails purity or origin tests; the bees' honey does not match the floral or regional profile claimed on the label.

The same pattern repeats with other so called "homemade" items. Big co-packing facilities might produce jams, jellies, and sauces. A vendor emails a recipe, wires a deposit, and the factory handles cooking, bottling, and labeling. The end product legally bears the vendor's brand but has never seen their stove. Unless you read the fine print on the back of the jar, you would never know.

Baked goods can be even more blatant. Some vendors buy cakes, cookies, pies, and bread from Costco, Sam's Club, or commercial bakeries. They peel off the plastic, slice or repackage them, and stack them under a gingham cloth labeled "homemade." A four dollar tray of cookies becomes a fifteen dollar "small batch" treat. Some go a step further: they re bake or drizzle icing over mass produced items to muddy the trail just enough to calm their conscience while keeping the markup.

Cheese is another playground for deception. True farmstead cheese, made from milk produced on the same farm where it is processed, is expensive to produce and often sells for fifteen to twenty dollars per pound or more. But a vendor can buy industrial cheese in bulk, cut it into wedges, wrap it in wax paper, and stick on a rustic label. Those same wedges can then be sold as "artisanal local cheese" for gourmet prices. Unless you are a trained taster or you know the actual producer, it is impossible to tell by sight alone.

Wholesale boxes and many individual produce items carry labels that identify the grower, packer, or country of origin. These stickers are the only physical link between what you are holding and its origin. The moment those labels are peeled off, the trail goes cold. Vendors can now claim, without fear of easy contradiction, "Yes, I grew that."

This is not just a moral problem; it is a food safety problem. If contamination occurs—a bad batch of melons, a pesticide residue issue, or a pathogen outbreak traceability matters. Supermarkets can review invoices and lot numbers. Your farmers' market vendor with a truck full of unlabeled produce cannot.

The situation becomes more ironic when customers assume "Amish" automatically means "organic" or chemical free. In reality, many Amish farms rely on conventional fertilizers and pesticides. Drive past an Amish auction, and you might see a truck parked near the horse drawn buggies, selling agricultural chemicals right out of the back. Some of these products are restricted use pesticides that require special licenses. Others are the same synthetic inputs used on large conventional farms. There are Amish farmers who use them, and resellers who later stand at the market claiming, "No sprays. All natural."

Layered on top of this local confusion is large scale organic fraud. Certification has become a multibillion dollar industry. When inspections are lax and enforcement is weak, the temptation to cheat grows. There have been documented cases of massive grain operations selling conventional crops as "organic" for years, pocketing millions in the process, and similar issues plague organic meat and dairy. Large confinement operations have secured organic labels while keeping animals indoors most of their lives, providing only token "access to pasture" to meet technical requirements.

From the customer's perspective, a carton of "organic" milk or a package of "grass fed, pasture raised" meat at a market table looks idyllic. But pictures of a green field on a sign do not guarantee that cows ever grazed there, or that chickens ever scratched in real dirt. In many industrial "organic" setups, a few animals are kept outside for photo and compliance purposes, while thousands remain inside on concrete floors. The marketing focuses on the handful in the sunshine.

You can see the same disconnect with sweet corn. That perfect, supermarket style ear—uniform size, bright yellow kernels, no worms, no chew marks—comes from treated or genetically engineered varieties. It is bred to look flawless and to resist pests, so it can be eaten raw right off the cob without any sign of damage.

Pesticide free or low spray corn often looks different. You might find a worm at the tip, a few ragged husk edges, or some uneven kernels. Farmers who avoid heavy chemicals accept that nature leaves a mark. Vendors promising "no chemicals ever" while selling boxes of flawless, identical ears week after week are not telling you the whole story.

At the heart of all this is simple arithmetic. Wholesale produce costs a fraction of what you pay at the farmers' market. If a vendor buys at half price and sells at triple price, the margins are enormous. A small reseller hitting several busy markets a week can clear a thousand dollars or more in profit without ever planting a seed or pulling a weed.

Real farming does not work that way. Real farmers shoulder land payments, seed costs, equipment debt, fuel, labor, weather risk, pests, and crop failures. Their profit margin per pound of produce is slim even in a good year. They cannot compete with someone who skips all of that and lives by "a van from the wholesale dock."

Market managers often lack both the authority and the resources to police this properly. Some markets do not ban reselling; they rely on honor systems and vague rules. State enforcement is patchy. A few places, like some parts of California and regions with producer only certifications, have stronger inspection programs, but many areas have little or no oversight. In that vacuum, the people who lie make the most money, and the honest ones disappear.

That is the real tragedy. The system, as it exists in many cities, rewards deception and punishes honesty. Genuine small farmers lose customers to cheaper, prettier fakes. Some quit the markets altogether, unable to keep up with prices or the endless, season defying variety of resellers. Does this mean every farmers' market is a scam? No. There are real farmers, real beekeepers, and real artisans still fighting to do things the right way. But in a system with weak enforcement and substantial financial incentives to cheat, blind trust is dangerous.

The only absolute protection is an educated, skeptical customer.

Chapter Twenty-Two

The Restaurant Won't Save You

RESTAURANTS, GHOST KITCHENS, AND institutional kitchens all run on the same industrial food system, no matter how pretty the plating or how pure the branding looks in the dining room.

Walking into a four star restaurant, the white tablecloths, cocktails, and potted herbs all signal safe and fresh, but what diners do not see are the walk in freezers, loading docks, and pallets of bulk food and food grade chemicals that make service possible. Most restaurants buy from the same large distributors that supply hospitals, stadiums, nursing homes, and fast food chains, not from small local farms for every item. Behind the swinging kitchen doors, trucks deliver industrial meat, fish, dairy, vegetables, and drums or bags of ingredients such as sodium tripolyphosphate, MSG, carrageenan, xanthan gum, and other emulsifiers, stabilizers, and preservatives designed to make food stable, uniform, and visually appealing across time and distance.

Those distributors are doing exactly what the modern food system rewards: supplying large volumes of consistent products that do not separate, spoil quickly, or change color while they sit in cold storage or on prep racks. To achieve that, many pre made sauces, glazes, marinades, and dressings come preloaded with thickeners, gums, dyes, and "processing aids" whose technical names never appear on restaurant menus. Sugar and salt are among the cheapest and most powerful tools in this toolbox, added generously because they make almost anything taste better; they also keep insulin and blood pressure working overtime when meals like this are a regular habit.

Take the classic "healthy" salmon dinner—grilled salmon, roasted potatoes, local corn, and a berry salad. The salmon is very often farmed Atlantic salmon raised in crowded sea pens on processed feed pellets rather than wild caught fish. Large surveys have found that farmed Atlantic salmon can carry higher average levels of PCBs and some organochlorine pollutants than certain wild salmon, enough that risk based consumption advisories have been issued in the past, even though modern feed changes have lowered some contaminant levels compared with earlier decades. Diners never see "polychlorinated biphenyls" written next to "lemon beurre blanc," and when a sugary glaze and salty rub are added, the dish can taste wonderful while quietly raising blood sugar and sodium intake.

The roasted potato typically comes from a large scale farm in major potato states, grown with synthetic fertilizers and protected with herbicides and fungicides to maximize yield and appearance; most diners cannot know whether that field saw glyphosate, chlorothalonil, or other pesticides. In many kitchens, "loaded" potatoes owe their flavor more to processed cheese sauces built from modified starches, emulsifiers, and artificial flavors than from simple cheese and cream. Corn served on the side in the United States almost always comes from genetically engineered varieties, since around 90 percent of U.S. corn acreage is planted in GMO hybrids, and restaurants generally buy affordable bulk bags rather than small batches of premium non GMO corn, often pre seasoned or pre sauced with added sugar and salt.

The side salad may wear a halo because of greens and berries, but the ingredients often travel far. Strawberries or blueberries can be imported from other hemispheres and moved through multiple packing houses, cold stores, and warehouses before reaching the kitchen, picking up handling and surface contamination risk at each stop. House dressings are frequently sweetened and salted enough that the "light" salad ends up rivaling sandwiches in sugar and sodium content, especially when creamy or fruit flavored. Unless a kitchen is unusually careful, cutting boards, sinks, and wiping cloths are common sources of cross contamination between raw and ready to eat foods, and inspections routinely find lapses even in reputable restaurants when sampling for bacteria on hands, gloves, rags, and equipment.

Ordering "healthy" premade dinners for delivery does not escape these dynamics. Many branded meals come from centralized commissary or ghost kitchens that the customer never sees; the brand on the app can be purely marketing. Ingredient lists often mirror processed foods: refined seed oils, gums such as xanthan or guar, modified starches, "natural flavors," and preservatives to keep texture and taste stable through chilling, shipping, and reheating. Sweet chili glazes, honey mustard sauces, and salted seasonings show up again and again because they are inexpensive and reliably enjoyable, not because they support metabolic health.

Fast food is simply the most overt expression of this system. Analyses of burgers and sandwiches from major chains show dozens of additives per item, including emulsifiers, thickeners, preservatives, colorants, and flavor enhancers, all optimized for deep freeze, rapid fry, and long hold times. Buns commonly include mono- and diglycerides and DATEM to keep them soft, while sauces rely on modified starches, EDTA, gums, and sweeteners to stay stable. Sugar appears in buns, sauces, and sometimes breadings, while sodium is heavily loaded into patties, cheese, fries, and coatings; engineered meals can meet minimum nutrition standards on paper but remain far from any traditional notion of simple, whole food.

Plant based or vegan restaurants are not automatically safer if they depend on the same distribution chain. Many rely on large produce wholesalers and broadline distributors for lettuce, peppers, tofu, and plant based meats that have travelled long distances. A convincing "veggie burger" often consists of isolated pea or soy protein, refined oils, methylcellulose, and complex flavor systems designed to mimic meat's texture and taste, making it an ultra processed food despite its vegan label. Vegan sauces and desserts can be heavy in sugar and salt because palates do not stop craving those tastes just because animal products are absent; "vegan" tells you what is not inside, but reveals little about pesticides, additives, or sodium levels.

Institutional settings such as nursing homes illustrate how budget and logistics shape food quality. Research in long term care facilities has found high rates of malnutrition or risk of malnutrition among residents, and studies evaluating menu quality conclude that average diet quality "could be improved," with pureed menus often lower in nutritional quality than regular texture menus. Facilities that rely heavily on commercially prepared pureed foods and heat-and-serve entrees tend to offer lower quality overall menus, with frequent use of gravies thickened by modified starches, reformed meats, pre packaged desserts, and "nutritional" shakes rich in added sugar and flavorings to encourage intake. These choices reflect cost and labor constraints more than optimal health.

The common thread across restaurants, ghost kitchens, fast food outlets, vegan cafés, and many nursing homes is that they source food from the same industrial universe: bulk meat, fish, eggs, produce, and grains from large suppliers plus catalogs of acids, gums, emulsifiers, colors, sweeteners, and preservatives to make everything cheaper, more stable, and more consistent. Citric and phosphoric acids, carrageenan and xanthan, polysorbates, titanium dioxide, high fructose corn syrup, sucralose, and many others are legal, widely used components of everyday dishes, even when they never appear on a printed menu. Salt and sugar remain the quiet co-stars, keeping flavor intensity high even when real ingredients are stretched thin.

When saying "the restaurant won't save you," the point is not that every chef is careless or every kitchen is dirty. The point is that the system they work in is built around bulk price, long shelf life, visual perfection, and repeatability, not around maximizing each diner's long term health. The more steps between a farm and a plate, and the more people and factories that season, pre cook, and decorate food, the more chances there are for nutrient loss, contamination, blood sugar spikes, and blood pressure surprises.

That does not mean never eating out; it means dropping the illusion that linen napkins, "artisan" on a menu, or a vegan icon magically erase these realities. Choosing simpler dishes with fewer mixed sauces, favoring grilled over breaded and fried, asking for dressings and sugary drinks on the side, and asking occasional questions about fish sources or cooking oils are practical ways to steer toward "less bad" options when dining out. Restaurants are entertainment and convenience first; nursing home trays and delivered meals are logistics solutions. For long term health, the unglamorous work of cooking most meals from recognizable ingredients at home still offers the most control. Treat every menu claim from "heart healthy" to "chef crafted" as marketing first and nutrition second, and let your own kitchen be the one place where the supply chain is not a black box.

Chapter Twenty-Three

Our Grocery Store Exit Plan: A New Way to Shop and Eat"

AVOIDING THE GROCERY STORE forever is not feasible, and blocking every chemical is not realistic. People will still need toilet paper, salt, beans, and a few things that only live under fluorescent lights. It is still possible to reduce the toxic dose and choose better options on each aisle by slowing down to read labels and reaching for the shortest, clearest ingredient lists on boxes, bottles, and jars, skipping walls of hard-to-say words in favor of foods your great-grandmother would recognize.

If you have reached the end of this book, you understand why relying only on grocery stores is not a healthy long-term plan. After pages of hidden hazards, the store can look like a minefield run by snack bandits. Avoiding it entirely is not possible, but there is a world of better options, some bold and some quiet, all safer, and this chapter serves as your roadmap to food freedom and practical damage control.

Modern health also depends on how time is spent each day. Hours lost to mindless television, extra errands, or nonessential chores could be invested in your food future: driving into the country, visiting small farm stands, or searching for local producers. You meet farmers who make cheese, milk, and butter without chemical shortcuts and who raise chickens, hogs, or cattle on real pasture instead of in crowded sheds, and you might plant stevia for sweetness in tea and cooking, turning your soil into a steady source of flavor and control.

Start by looking at yards. People spend billions maintaining tens of millions of acres of lawn that absorb chemicals, fuel, and water and yield nothing in return, while the easiest win is to rip out part of that grass and plant something edible. Urban agriculture projects show that an average home garden can produce hundreds of dollars' worth of vegetables and herbs each year, and community gardeners often grow twice the yield per square foot as large farms, though the work is hands-on and steady.

Instead of filling every corner of your yard with ornamentals, turn some of that space into a living spice cabinet. Herbs like chamomile and mint grow quickly and yield multiple harvests each season, providing soothing teas and bright flavor for almost no cost. Add cooking herbs such as basil, oregano, thyme, rosemary, and parsley, and you suddenly have the backbone of every soup, sauce, and roast just steps from your door, ready to dry in a simple dehydrator and grind into clean, powerful seasonings.

Kitchen "scraps" can become tools, not trash. Garlic scapes, onion tops, carrot peels, celery leaves, and similar trimmings dry well and blend into your own vegetable broth mix, ready to scoop into winter soups and stews. There are no complex rules;

you build an arsenal of herbs and spices that match your taste instead of a factory formula, and each jar replaces a chemical-laced blend with something you grow, dry, and trust yourself. Over time, your pantry turns into a quiet apothecary of flavor and medicine.

You can find a farmer who raises real birds for meat and hogs, lambs, and cattle that live on pasture rather than concrete. Instead of buying one package at a time, you buy a larger share and turn your kitchen into a small preservation shop, using a pressure canner to fill glass jars with meat, broth, and herbs, processing 20 quarts at once into ready-to-heat dinners. Those jars rest on pantry shelves for years, ready for busy nights, while extra vegetables slide into jars and overflowing tomatoes head for the freezer for sauces, soups, and stews.

With a sturdy pressure canner, a water-bath pot for jams and jellies, and tough tools like a grinder, food processor, and breadmaker, you transform clean animals and produce into jerky, sausage, stocks, and preserves. You control salt, fat, and spices and avoid pesticides, dyes, and artificial preservatives, and every jar becomes a small investment in your health instead of a profit center for a distant factory, building a wall of insurance against storms, shortages, and long workdays.

Beverages deserve the same scrutiny because they are a hidden trap. Bottled and canned teas often contain only a fraction of the antioxidants in homemade tea and are high in sugar and preservatives, while backyard herbal teas from mint, lemon balm, or sage can pour flavor straight from a home garden. Homemade iced tea takes about a minute and delivers taste, plant compounds, and no microplastics, making brewing at home or infusing water with herbs and lemon slices the safe, simple move.

When you cannot grow enough yourself, go directly. Farmers' markets continue to expand, and Community Supported Agriculture programs let you buy a share of a farm's harvest, sending money straight to real people instead of distant corporations. Every box of vegetables that arrives from a CSA skips weeks of storage, long truck rides, and towering stacks of plastic, and the safest, healthiest pattern is to eat what grows in season near your home, mostly unwrapped.

Bulk buying clubs and co-ops help neighborhoods save money and support local makers. Co-ops draw in members who want clean meals, clear labels, and stronger communities, often support small farms, donate locally, and favor ingredients that are easy to pronounce, while giving members discounts and a real say in what appears on shelves; joining one lets you sidestep the worst packaging and mystery ingredients without giving up pleasure.

Cooking at home is the strongest safety measure you have. Industrial processing strips nutrients and pours in salt, sugar, and preservatives, while home-cooked meals usually taste better and cost less per serving, especially when cooked in batches. Fermenting or pickling garden produce strengthens gut health and can help lower risk for several chronic conditions, and home canning fills pantries with glass jars instead of lined cans, turning potential waste into dependable meals.

Snack swaps deliver immediate benefits. Instead of a plastic-wrapped cake with a long label, you bake with flour, eggs, and honey and taste every ingredient, or you pop your own popcorn, dry extra apples, or roast nuts for clean, fast snacks. For energy on the go, you mix granola or roll oat balls at home and avoid artificial dyes and sugar spikes—choosing to prepare snacks yourself or buy fruit and nuts instead of grabbing them off a factory wall.

Sharing and bartering magnify these gains. Food swaps let people trade herb pesto for jam, beans for hot sauce, or eggs for handmade bread at libraries, churches, parks, and neighborhood events, shifting focus from money to what you grow, make, or bake. Hosting or joining a swap, or just knocking on a neighbor's door with extra soup or zucchini, builds safety and connection one dish at a time.

If you live in a city without a yard, community gardening opens new doors. Urban garden programs now number in the thousands, with shared plots and millions of gardeners tending small beds; many sites match you with space, water, tools, and even seeds or starter plants. You can also grow in containers on balconies, permitted fire escapes, or sunny windowsills, making the safest, healthiest move to claim any available space and turn it into food.

When you return to the store, act like a label detective. Skip products with long ingredient lists and vague "flavor" words that hide unknown blends, aim to eat with the seasons, and use bulk bins for beans, lentils, nuts, seeds, and oats from places that rotate stock often. The safer choice is to favor loose, lightly packaged foods with fewer steps between farm and plate.

For protein, look beyond the giant meat case. Seek local butchers, egg farms, and fish counters that answer questions about source, feed, and living conditions, asking how animals live, what they eat, and how often deliveries arrive. Look for pasture-raised, grass-fed, and wild-caught options that fit your budget, and visit farms or docks when possible to see how that protein begins its journey.

Rethink storage at home as well. Glass and stainless steel are the best containers because they do not shed microplastics or off-flavors, and avoiding single-use plastic and never microwaving in plastic reduces exposure and waste. Reusable containers, cloth covers, and beeswax wraps protect flavor and leftovers while cutting trash, giving you boxes and jars you can wash, reuse, and trust for years.

Old habits are hard to break, but each small change trims your grocery bill and your health risks. Growing mint, splitting a CSA box, or joining a food swap gradually builds new routines that feel normal, and perfection is never the goal. Each yard, kitchen, and shared table becomes a little more aligned with your values and biology; the healthiest food stays close to your hands, your dirt, and your neighbors' tables, not at the far end of a delivery truck.

Whenever you return to the aisles, remember your role. You are not just a customer under bright lights with a cart; you are a grower, a cook, a swapper, a preserver, and a builder of sturdy habits around real food. Your quiet revolution begins with a shovel, a jar, and a recipe on a worn card or screen, and as seasons pass, you eat well, live stronger, and enjoy a little more freedom with every harvest and every shared meal.

Chapter Twenty-Four

Glossary of Grocery Store Ingrediency

3-MCPD: Chemical contaminant formed during oil refining, especially bleaching or high-heat deodorizing. Toxic to kidneys and may promote cancer. Found at low levels in many processed foods and oils.

Acephate: Insecticide used on crops like green beans and peppers. Works by attacking insects' nervous systems. Long-term exposure harms human nerves and kidneys.

Acesulfame Potassium (Ace-K): Calorie-free artificial sweetener, 200 times sweeter than sugar. Blended with other sweeteners for taste and used in diet sodas, sweets, and protein powders.

Acrylamide: Chemical produced when coffee beans or foods are roasted at high temperatures; linked to nerve damage and is considered a probable human carcinogen.

Acrylates: Synthetic plastic films, not natural, can irritate the gut and immune system.

Additives: Substances added to drinks, processed foods, or condiments for appearance, texture, flavor, or shelf life. Includes preservatives or stabilizers; can cause allergic or digestive reactions.

Advantame: High-intensity sweetener, about 20,000 times sweeter than sugar. Recently approved, chemically similar to aspartame, with uncertain long-term effects.

Aflatoxin: Mold toxin produced by fungi on animal feed, and can pass into milk, wheat, or cheese. Potent liver carcinogen.

Aldehyde: Toxic byproduct formed when vegetable oil is heated. Damages cells/DNA, linked to cancer and heart disease risk.

Aluminum Compounds (Sodium Aluminum Phosphate, etc.): Used as leavening agents, produced from aluminum and sodium salts. Regular intake may harm the nervous system and kidneys.

Ammonia: Used in food processing and can cleaning solutions to break down proteins and sterilize. Irritates lungs and digestive tract, especially in high concentrations.

Ammonium Nitrate: Powerful synthetic fertilizer, used to boost fruit size/yield; overuse disrupts soil and plant nutrition, build-up contaminates water.

Amoxicillin: Antibiotic given to cows for infections, residues remain in milk if not withdrawn correctly. Can cause allergies and promote drug resistance.

Annatto/Annatto Extract: Natural orange-yellow coloring from seeds, used in cheese/butter. Rarely allergenic, unnecessary in pure dairy.

Antibiotics: Drugs used to treat infections (often for animals/cows), residues end up in food, can trigger resistance/allergies.

Antimony/Antimony Trioxide: Toxic metal used in PET plastics, carcinogenic if leached into food/water; disrupts hormones and organ function.

Anti-caking Agent (Silicon Dioxide, Calcium Silicate): Prevents spice mixes from clumping. Usually safe in small amounts, may dilute nutrition if used excessively.

Artificial Colors: Dyes made from petroleum distillates, cause allergies, hyperactivity, and may increase cancer risk.

Artificial Flavors: Synthetic chemicals created in labs to mimic real food taste, can upset digestion, trigger allergies, and offer no nutrition.

Aspartame: Artificial sweetener, 200 times sweeter than sugar; linked to headaches, brain issues, and some cancer risks.

Atrazine: Herbicide sprayed on grain crops and feed, disrupts hormones, linked with fertility trouble, contaminates dairy/meat via animal consumption.

Azo Dye: Synthetic chemical dyes, bright red/orange/yellow, some linked to hyperactivity, allergies, cancer risk.

Azodicarbonamide: Chemical used as a dough conditioner/bleaching agent, banned in EU/Australia for links to asthma/cancer.

Azoxystrobin: Fungicide applied to apples, grapes, and berries; residue can irritate the gut.

Baking Soda: Chemically produced from soda ash. Used as a leavening agent, can cause bloating and disrupt stomach acid if overused.

Bamboo Shoots: Harvested immature bamboo, peeled and canned, treated with acid/salt for texture; high sodium/low nutrition.

Barley: Cooked, peeled, pressure-processed grains lose fiber/nutrients, can spike blood sugar.

Beef Broth: Factory-processed bones/tissue boiled down, may contain hormone, antibiotic, and contaminant residues.

Beet Sugar: Sugar derived from beets, chemically similar to cane sugar, lacks natural nutrients.

Beta-Agonists (e.g., ractopamine): Growth drugs for pigs/cattle; banned in most places due to links with heart and nervous issues.

BHA (Butylated Hydroxyanisole): Synthetic antioxidant preservative, disrupts hormones, possible carcinogen, banned or restricted in many nations.

BHT (Butylated Hydroxytoluene): Synthetic antioxidant preservative, keeps oils stable, impacts hormones, possible cancer risk.

Bisphenol A/Bisphenol S/BPA/BPS: Chemical hardeners in packaging/plastics, leach hormones, fertility, development disruptors.

Bleach/Bleached Flour: Chemical treatment for produce/packaging and flour whitening, damages cells/nutrition.

Blue 1: Synthetic dye from petroleum, may trigger allergic reactions/hyperactivity.

Botulism/Cronobacter: Deadly bacteria that can contaminate baby foods/formula, causes vomiting, paralysis, and can be fatal, especially for infants.

Bran: Fiber-rich layer of wheat kernel, removed in white flour milling.

Bread: Packaged with preservatives and slip agents, often made from refined flour, sugar, and artificial flavors; long shelf life, gut/hormone irritants.

Brown Sugar Syrup: Refined cane or beet sugar mixed with molasses; causes blood sugar spikes.

Butterfat: Fat part of milk/cream, stores contaminants, raises flavor (and risk factors).

Byproducts: All non-prime muscles and organ scraps ground into processed meats and pet food; higher residue/additive content.

Cadmium: Heavy metal contaminant from fertilizer, soil, irrigation runoff; harms kidneys, bones, can cause cancer.

Calcium Carbonate: Mineral ground for calcium supplements, overuse blocks absorption/stresses kidneys.

Calcium Chloride: Preserves texture in canned produce, high amounts disrupt calcium in diet.

Calcium Phosphate/Monocalcium/Dicalcium Phosphate: Added to foods, disrupt mineral balance in excess.

Calcium Propionate: Preservative, disrupts gut bacteria and digestion.

Cane Sugar: Extracted/refined sugar, calories only, spikes blood sugar.

Caramel Color: Formed by heating sugars, can contain ammonia byproducts linked to cancer.

Carnauba Wax: Palm leaf wax in fruit coatings, edible but traps pesticide residues.

Carrageenan: Seaweed-derived thickener, heavily processed, known to cause gut irritation/allergies in sensitive people.

Captan: Fungicide for apples/berries, irritates skin/gut on exposure.

Carbaryl: Insecticide for apples/greens, blocks nerve impulses, can affect humans at high doses.

Cellulose Gum/Xanthan Gum: Thickeners from plant fermentation, may disrupt digestion/promote unhealthy bacterial growth.

Cheese: Factory processed with salt, enzymes, anti-caking agents, wrapped in plastics, absorbs contaminants and coloring, can increase cancer risk and disrupt hormones.

Chlorine Dioxide: Flour bleach, leaves residue, banned in some countries.

Chlorine Wash: Meat and produce processors use chlorine to kill bacteria, disrupts gut microbiome.

Chlorpyrifos: Pesticide, banned other places but still used here; harms brain development and memory.

Citric Acid: Acidulant from industrial fermentation, not real fruit, can erode teeth/cause digestive issues.

Citrus Red 2: Synthetic dye, enhances orange peel, banned in some places for cancer risk.

Colorants: Industrial pigments in foods, allergies/hyperactivity/cancer risk.

Condiments: Processed sauces (e.g., ketchup/mayo/mustard); high sugar, starch, preservatives, bottled in plastics.

Corn/Corn Starch/Modified Corn Starch: Canned/processed, loses nutrients, spikes blood sugar, often contains GMOs.

Cream-Filled Pastry: Baked goods with dairy/egg filling, risk microbial contamination.

Cross Contamination: Mixing of allergens, toxins, or foreign substances during processing; triggers severe allergic reactions.

DDT: Banned insecticide, long soil/fat persistence, causes hormone/cancer/development problems.

DEHA: Plasticizer in packaging, disrupts hormones.

Dextrose: Corn sweetener, calorie-only, spikes blood sugar.

Diced Tomatoes: Processed/peeled/pasteurized, lined with plastics/acids.

Diphenylamine (DPA): Preservative for apple skin, breakdown irritates tissues.

Disodium EDTA: Stabilizer, bioaccumulates, disrupts minerals.

Dithiocarbamates: Fungicide, thyroid risk.

Dough Conditioner: Chemicals (azodicarbonamide/L-cysteine) for dough/baking, trigger allergies, not from food sources.

DNA Barcoding: Genetic ID for seafood; inconsistent use allows fraud/contamination.

Emulsifier: Chemicals to blend ingredients (mono/diglycerides/soy lecithin), disrupt gut, trigger allergies/sensitivities.

Enrichment: Synthetic vitamins/iron added to flour after milling.

Epoxy Resin: Petrochemical packaging coating migrates into food, disrupts hormones.

Erucamide: Slip agent for bags, long-term effects unknown.

Ethyl Butyrate: Synthetic frozen juice flavor pack ingredient, gut/respiratory irritant.

Extraction Rate: Percent of flour from grain after milling; lower rate means less nutrition.

FDA (Food and Drug Administration): Regulates bottled water, less stringent than EPA for tap water.

Feed (Aquafeed): GMO/chemical-laden feed for fish and animals; contaminant risk.

Festival Treat: Sweet/high-fat snacks, colorful, loosely regulated.

Filtration: Water treatment, may not remove microplastics/PFAS/metals.

Finely Textured Beef ("Pink Slime"): Meat filler spun from beef scraps, treated with ammonia/citric acid, pathogen risk.

Flavor Packs: Engineered blends of aroma chemicals added to juice (e.g., orange), not present in fresh juice, unknown health effects.

Fludioxonil: Fungicide for berries/melons/greens; residue can impact gut health.

Formaldehyde: Chemical disinfectant/preservative, damages nerves, carcinogenic.

Forever Chemicals (PFAS): Persistent toxins found in food/water/packaging, disrupt hormones/immunity/cancer risk.

Frozen Dough/Premix: Factory-mixed dough with preservatives.

Fruit/Fruit Cocktail: Canned/blanched fruit in syrup/acids, loses nutrients/gains contaminants from packaging.

Gene Editing: DNA modification in wheat, rarely studied for human safety.

Gelling Agents: Thicken/stabilize foods, may be non-organic in "organic" labeled products.

Glutamate: Amino acid added as MSG, may overstimulate nerves/symptoms.

Glucono Delta-Lactone: Fermented glucose acidulant, alters gut flora/taste when consumed in excess.

Glyphosate: Herbicide for wheat/produce, cancer risk, disrupts gut health.

Glycidol: Oil processing byproduct, proven carcinogen, most present in processed oils/fried food.

Green Beans: Canned/processed with salt/firms, loses nutrients.

Growth Hormones: Synthetic animal hormones, disrupt human hormones/cancer risk.

Guar Gum: Bean-derived thickener for cheese/dairy/yogurt, large amounts disrupt gut/mineral absorption.

Heavy Metals (Lead, Cadmium, Mercury, Arsenic): Toxic elements from soil/packaging/foods, damage tissues/nerves/kidneys/child development.

Hearts of Palm: Pre-boiled/canned, salty, bland, shelf-stable.

Herbicide: Chemical weed killers, residue persists in tea/coffee; cancer/hormone risk.

Hexane: Petroleum oil extraction solvent, traces can remain toxic, not nutritious.

High Fructose Corn Syrup (HFCS): Sweetener from corn starch, blood sugar spike, linked to obesity and diabetes.

Honey, Fake or Adulterated: Mixed with other syrups, lacks enzymes/minerals.

Hydrogenation: Adds hydrogens to oil to make trans fats, raises heart/inflammatory disease risk.

Hydrolyzed Protein: Proteins broken down, flavor enhancer, triggers allergies.

IGF-1 (Insulin-like Growth Factor 1): Hormone raised by rBGH in cows, tied to possible cancer risks.

Imidacloprid: Neurotoxic pesticide for fruit/veg/citrus; disrupts bees/pollinators.

Interesterified Fat: Lab-mixed fats to replace trans fats, alters sugar metabolism, unknown long-term risk.

Invert Sugar: Syrup sweeter than sugar, used in confectionary/baked goods.

Iron (Fortified): Lab-created iron salt added to foods, excess is irritating to the gut.

Jackfruit: Canned tropical fruit, processed with brine, low in nutrients.

L-cysteine: Amino acid used for dough, can come from hair or feathers, linked to allergies/digestion issues.

Lead: Metal contaminant, impairs brain development, linked to chronic health harms.

Leavening Agents: Baking powder/soda blends to make foods rise; overuse disrupts electrolytes/gut balance.

Linoleic Acid: Main omega-6 fatty acid, excess risk for obesity/cancer/heart risk.

Lotus Root: Sliced/canned in saline, crunchy, low nutrition, high sodium.

Lychees: Canned in syrup/acids, high sugar, less nutritional than fresh.

Maltodextrin: Starch-based sweetener/binder for low-cal foods, spikes blood sugar.

Margarine: Made from processed oils, linked to inflammation/heart disease.

Maneb: Fungicide for celery/potatoes/tomatoes, affects nerves/thyroid.

Maraschino dye (Red 40, Red 3): For cherries/cocktails, risk allergies/behavioral effects.

Mechanically Separated Chicken/Pork: Pressed scraps with phosphate fillers, not real muscle, starchy and chemical-laden.

Mercury: Toxic metal, accumulates in predator fish, causes nerve/brain damage.

Methamidophos: Insecticide/fungicide, banned many places, damages nerves, found in some produce.

Methylene Chloride: Solvent for decaf coffee, probable carcinogen if trace remains.

Milk Fat: Industrially extracted fat, high in saturated fat and risk for inflammation/heart disease.

Milk (and non-dairy): Ultra-pasteurized/processed, bottled with plastics, loses live cultures and nutrients, packaging chemicals leach in over time.

Milling: Wheat crushing process, removes bran/germ for less nutritious flour.

Microplastics: Tiny synthetic fragments from packaging, found in beverages, dairy, seafood, and formula. Health effects are uncertain.

Mono- and Diglycerides: Manufactured fats/emulsifiers, disrupt metabolism/inflammation.

Monoglycerides/Diglycerides: Used for blending fats in bread/dairy; alter cholesterol/fat absorption.

Monk Fruit Sweetener: Highly processed extract, very sweet, usually blended with other sweeteners.

Morpholine: Chemical in wax coatings for produce/dairy, reacts with nitrites to form nitrosamines, carcinogenic when mixed.

Natural Flavor: Lab-engineered blend of animal and plant extracts, processed with solvents. Hidden additives may cause allergies or sensitivities.

Niacinamide: Synthesized vitamin B3 used for fortification. Excess can damage the liver but rarely offers the same benefit as food-based vitamins.

Norovirus and Hepatitis: Viruses often found in shellfish raised or harvested from polluted waters. Infection causes severe illness; not present in wild, unpolluted seafood.

Nuts and Snack Bags: Salted, roasted, and preserved with BHT, then sealed in multilayer pouches (PET, foil, polypropylene). Roasted nuts lose nutrients and absorb plastic residues. Snack mixes often contain high salt, sugar, and preservatives, increasing cancer, heart, and gut risk.

Omega-3/Omega-6: Fats from fish/flax/walnuts and seed oils; anti-inflammatory omega-3 is under-consumed. Omega-6 excess found in processed foods fuels inflammation.

Olives: Soaked in brine, lye, and color stabilizers. Often high in salt and missing beneficial raw nutrients or live cultures.

Onions: Dehydrated, chopped, pressure cooked in synthetic broth. Minimal nutrition and flavor lost in heat.

Palm Oil: Extracted and refined from palm fruit, usually high heat and chemicals. Raises saturated fat and is linked to deforestation and heart disease risk.

Parabens: Chemical antimicrobials used in packaging. Linked to cancer and hormone problems.

Peaches: Blanched, peeled, and canned in syrup, with added color and acid. High in sugar, fewer vitamins than fresh.

Pear: Blanched, peeled, cooked in heavy syrup. Mostly texture, sugar, little nutrition.

Peas: Pre-cooked, canned in salt, firmed with chemicals. Lose vitamins C and B, loaded with sodium.

PFAS (Per- and Polyfluoroalkyl Substances): Persistent "forever chemicals" found in water, food and some produce packaging; tied to cancer, immune issues, hormone changes.

Phosphates: Synthetic chemicals injected into foods (meat, seafood, bakery) to boost moisture/content/yield. Raise sodium burden and can strain kidneys/bones.

Phthalates: Plastics softeners in food packaging, migrate into food over time. Endocrine disruptors linked to infertility and development issues.

Pineapple: Blanched, cored, canned in heavy syrup/juice. Loses enzymes, spikes blood sugar.

Plasticizers (Phthalates, BPA, BPS, Vinyl Chloride, Styrene): Chemicals that leach from can/package walls and disrupt hormone, immune, developmental health.

Polyethylene/Polypropylene/Polystyrene/PVC: Synthetic plastics used in food boxes for durability or sealing. Leach hormone-disrupting chemicals under certain conditions.

Polyphosphates: Synthetic preservative chemicals to lock water and texture "fresh." Damage kidneys, may lower bone over time.

Pork Fat: Rendered, cooked, added for "mouthfeel." Increases saturated fat and shelf life, not nutrition.

Potassium Bromate: Added to commercial flour, banned in many countries due to its link to cancer, still found in US processed bread.

Potassium Sorbate: Preservative in fruit/pie fillings, inhibits yeast/mold, excessive intake can cause irritation.

Preservatives (Propyl Gallate, Sodium Stearoyl Lactylate, Sodium Benzoate, Sodium Diacetate, Potassium Acetate, Sodium Metabisulfite, Sorbic Acid): Synthetic chemicals prolong shelf life, can provoke allergies, digestive issues, and even carcinogens when combined with other chemicals.

Propylene Glycol (Mono/Diesters): Synthetic byproducts (plastic-making); smooth texture in foods. May harm kidneys, liver over time.

Pumpkin: Cooked, pureed, canned with stabilizers. Most fiber and vitamin A survives; other nutrients diminish.

Pyrethroids: Lab-synthesized insecticides used for agriculture, found on frozen vegetables. Known to trigger allergies and disrupt nerves/hormones.

Radioactive Contaminants: Isotopes from nuclear accidents found in ocean/lake ecosystems and migratory fish; pose long-term health risks.

Ractopamine: Beta-agonist drug added to pig/cattle feed to increase muscle, banned in most countries, causes heart/muscle/behavioral issues.

Red 40/Red 3/Erythrosine: Petroleum-based dyes banned in some nations, linked to allergies, hyperactivity, cancer/thyroid risks.

Rendered Fat: Made by melting/processing animal scraps leftover from slaughter; high in saturated fat, may have chemicals.

Salt: Highly processed, purified, stripped of minerals. Excessive amounts harm blood pressure and heart.

Sardines: Gutted and canned whole in oil/sauce. Sometimes contain mercury or contaminants from environment.

Scombroid Poisoning: Foodborne illness from improperly refrigerated tuna/mackerel, causes toxic histamine buildup, triggers allergic/cardiovascular symptoms.

Smoke Flavor: Real smoke condensed, processed, recombined. Linked to gut irritation, little nutritional value.

Sodium Benzoate: Chemical preservative; can form carcinogenic benzene with vitamin C, worsen allergies.

Sodium Hydroxide: Powerful industrial base—peels/cleans vegetables/cans; traces damage gut/cells.

Sodium Nitrite/Nitrate: Preserves pinkness in meats, forms nitrosamines (carcinogenic) when cooked at high temps.

Sodium Phosphate: Used in boxed cheese, upsets mineral balance, strains kidneys/bones.

Soy Lecithin/Soybean Oil: Processed fats from soybeans used in foods; can cause allergies and gut disruption, high in omega-6 promotes inflammation.

Spinach: Canned, blanched, chopped, canned with salt or acid. Most vitamins lost, sodium remains high.

Styrene: Plastic and can lining chemical, leaches in small quantities; suspected carcinogen/disrupts cell function.

Sugar: Refined from cane/beets, filtered to white crystals. Drives up obesity, diabetes, heart disease, tooth problems.

Sunflower Oil/Canola Oil/Vegetable Oil: Chemically extracted and processed at high heat. Easily oxidizes, fuels artery inflammation.

Sucralose (Artificial Sweeteners): Lab-created sweeteners, zero calories, alter gut bacteria, may increase weight/insulin issues.

TBHQ (Tertiary Butylhydroquinone): Preservative from butane, harms immune system, linked to allergies/cancer risk.

Thiabendazole: Fungicide for bananas/citrus, high exposures linked to liver/thyroid damage.

Titanium Dioxide: Mined, purified, used for whitening foods. May damage DNA, controversial safety at high doses.

Trans Fats/Partially Hydrogenated Oils: Made by injecting hydrogen into oil. Damages cholesterol, increases inflammation, heart disease risk.

Transglutaminase (Meat Glue): Enzyme manufactured from bacteria or animal sources; binds meat pieces, not natural, pathogen risk.

Tripotassium Phosphate: Synthetic mineral salt found in boxed cereals/noodles. Weakens bones, irritates kidneys, promotes inflammation.

Tuna: Cooked, packed in water/brine/oil. May contain mercury, sodium, factory wash residues.

Vanillin (Artificial Vanilla): Synthesized from wood pulp or petrochemicals. Flavor lacks nutrition, can trigger headaches/allergies.

Vegetable Oil: Extracted, refined from plants with chemicals, linked to inflammation/heart risk.

Vinyl Chloride: Plasticizer in can coatings, linked to liver toxicity and cancer.

Water: Used as filler/cooking medium in canned food, can contain dissolved preservatives/minerals, dilutes nutrients.

Wheat Flour: Refined, bleached before canning. Loses fiber, raises blood sugar, loses vitamins.

Whey: Cheese byproduct, dehydrated for processed food, may upset digestion, less nutritious than whole dairy.

Wild-caught: Seafood fished from natural habitats, lower contaminant risk than factory farmed, but still vulnerable to environmental pollution.

Xanthan Gum: Thickener made by bacterial fermentation of sugars, high doses may cause bloating/gas.

Yeast Extract: Created by breaking down yeast with heat/chemicals, salty flavor enhancer, can cause reactions in sensitive people.

Yellow 6: Synthetic orange dye from petroleum, banned in some places, allergy/cancer.

Chapter Twenty-Five

Bibliography

CHAPTER I: FRANKEN FOOD Fiesta: The Boxed Food Trap

Anderson Cancer Center. (2023). 7 Examples of Processed Food. Retrieved from **https://mdanderson.org**

BHF. (2025). Ultra-Processed Foods: How Bad Are They for Your Health? British Heart Foundation. Retrieved from **https://bhf.org.uk**

Consumer Reports. (2022). Dangerous PFAS Chemicals Are in Your Food Packaging. Retrieved from **https://consumerreports.org**

Duke Recreation. (2024). Keeping it Simple: A Guide for Grocery Shopping. Retrieved from **https://recreation.duke.edu**

Epicurious. (2017). The Best "Healthy" Boxed Cake Mixes. Retrieved from **https://epicurious.com**

FoodPrint. (2020). Chemicals in Food Packaging. Retrieved from **https://foodprint.org**

GoodFoodFighter. (2019). Supermarket Bakeries: Please Stop Using Cancer-Causing Ingredients. Retrieved from **https://goodfoodfighter.com**

Health Digest. (2022). The Truth About What's Really In Pancake Mix. Retrieved from **https://healthdigest.com**

Healthline. (2022). The Sweet Danger of Sugar. Retrieved from **https://health.harvard.edu**

Healthline. (2023). Are Instant Noodles Bad for You? Retrieved from **https://healthline.com**

Mayo Clinic Press. (2024). Key Ingredients to Avoid in Ultra Processed Foods. Retrieved from **https://mcpress.mayoclinic.org**

MD Anderson Cancer Center. (2023). 7 Examples of Processed Food. Retrieved from **https://mdanderson.org**

NIH PMC. (2018). The Hidden Dangers of Fast and Processed Food. Retrieved from **https://pmc.ncbi.nlm.nih.gov**

Nutrition Source, Harvard. (2025). Processed Foods and Health. Retrieved from **https://nutritionsource.hsph.harvard.edu**

Parkwayeast.com.sg. (2024). How Bad Are Instant Noodles for Your Health? Retrieved from **https://parkwayeast.com.sg**

PFAS Free UK. (2025). PFAS in Food Packaging. Retrieved from **https://pfasfree.org.uk**

Pillsbury. (2025). Ready to Bake! Chick Shape Sugar Cookie Dough. Retrieved from **https://pillsbury.com**

Stanford Medicine. (2025). Ultra-Processed Food: Five Things to Know. Retrieved from **https://med.stanford.edu**

Toxic-Free Future. (2025). Toxic Chemicals in Food Packaging: PFAS, Phthalates, and Other Chemicals. Retrieved from **https://toxicfreefuture.org**

UC Davis. (2025). What to Know About Processed and Ul-

tra-Processed Food. Retrieved from **https://ucdavis.edu**
Vovk, M. (2025). PFAS: The Forever Chemicals Poisoning Water, People and Wildlife. [Book reference for PFAS section]
WebMD. (2023). Healthiest Flour for Baking. Retrieved from **https://webmd.com**
Yale Medicine. (2025). Are Ultraprocessed Foods Bad for Your Health? Retrieved from **https://yalemedicine.org**

Chapter 2: Canned Carnage: The Poison Parade in Every Pantry

BCPP. (2024). Food Packaging Chemicals. Breast Cancer Prevention Partners.
BMJ. (2023). Food additive emulsifiers and risk of cardiovascular disease in the NutriNet-Santé cohort: Prospective cohort study.
Center for Environmental Health. (2020). Canned Foods.
Harvard Health Publishing. (2021). Common food additives and chemicals harmful to children.
Healthline. (2019). Canned Food: Good or Bad?
Mayo Clinic. (2023). What is BPA? Should I be worried about it?
National Institutes of Health. (2022). Toxicological and teratogenic effect of various food additives.
PubMed. (2024). Artificial food additives: Hazardous to long-term health?
Scientific American. (2015). BPA still widely used in canned goods.
Stanford Medicine. (2016). Study shows link between canned

food, exposure to hormone disruptor BPA.
U.S. Department of Agriculture. (Various years). National Center for Home Food Preservation.
University Hospitals. (2025). Should you be concerned about food additives?
Washington Post. (2025). Avoid these 5 food additives that may harm your health.
WHO. (2023). Food additives—World Health Organization.
Yale Medicine. (Various years). Processed foods and health: Sources and risks.

Chapter 3: Plastic Wrap Roulette: Eating Food in a Toxic Tomb

Beyond Plastics. (2024). Cheese packaged in plastic may expose you to harmful chemicals.
Breast Cancer Prevention Partners. (2024). Food packaging chemicals.
Capital Resin Corporation. (2025). 7 types of plastic packaging for food.
Center for Environmental Health. (2024). Toxic ingredients in food packaging.
ChemTrust. (2024). Harmful chemicals from plastics found in popular US supermarket foods.
Consumer Reports. (2024). The plastic chemicals hiding in your food.
Food Packaging Forum. (2024). Report finds harmful chemicals widespread in packaged and supermarket foods.
Healthline. (2019). 12 common food additives—Should you

avoid them?
Kitchen Stories. (2025). Experts warn: Eating from plastic containers can harm your health.
Lacerta Group. (2025). The thermoforming plastic packaging process, explained.
Mayo Clinic Press. (2024). Key ingredients to avoid in ultra processed foods.
National Institutes of Health. (2024). Plastic products leach chemicals that induce in vitro toxicity.
NPR. (2024). Chemicals from food packaging leach into food—affecting people's health.□
O.Berk. (2025). Plastic containers manufacturing process.
PMC-NIH. (2021). Plastic food container safety.
SafetyCulture. (2025). Food packaging manufacturing: A guide.
Toxic-Free Future. (2025). Toxic chemicals in food packaging: PFAS, phthalates, and other chemicals.
U.S. EPA. (2025). Containers and packaging: Product-specific data.
Wise Owl Lifestyle. (2025). Health risks of plastic food containers: Heating & freezing concerns.

Chapter 4: Iced Deceit: The Chilling Truth About Frozen Grocery Food

Blogs.IFAS.UFL.edu. (2021). Grocery shopping for your health: The freezer section.
Center for Science in the Public Interest. (2025). The cold, hard

facts about frozen foods.
Chefs for Seniors. (2024). Hidden dangers of grocery store frozen meals.
Eat This, Not That! (2025). 11 unhealthiest frozen dinners you should avoid.
FDA. (2025). 2025 recalls of prepared pasta meals (frozen and ready-to-eat foods).
Good Morning America. (2011). Orange juice's 'secret' flavor packet surprises some moms.□
GoodRx. (2025). 6 U.S. food ingredients that are banned abroad.
Newsweek. (2025). These food additives in your US food are banned in Europe—See the list.
The Nutrition Insider. (2025). Red flag ingredients: Food additives to avoid in frozen food.
University of Utah Health. (2025). The truth about frozen food.
Yale Medicine. (2025). Are ultra processed foods bad for your health?

Chapter 5: Behind the Meat Counter: Factories, Fillers, and Health Risks

Animal Welfare Institute. (2024). Inhumane practices on factory farms.
ASPCA. (2023). Factory farming: A recipe for disaster for animals & our planet.
Center for Food Safety. (2025). The truth about factory-farmed

meat in the U.S.
CIWF (Compassion in World Farming). (2025). Health impacts of factory farming on people.
Earth Day Network. (2025). The cruel costs of factory farming.
Food Revolution Network. (2023). The truth about grassfed beef.
Healthline. (2019). Grass-fed vs. grain-fed beef—What's the difference?□
National Cattle Comfort. (2020). Antibiotics, hormones, and feed additives.
NIH. (2025). Impact of genetically modified organisms on meat quality.
ScienceDirect. (2014). Meat byproducts—An overview.
USDA. (2025). Animal production.
World Animal Protection. (2025). Factory farming statistics you need to know.
World Animal Protection. (2025). Hidden health impacts of factory farming.
Yale Medicine. (2025). Are ultra processed foods bad for your health?

Chapter 6: Poisoned Catch: The Truth About Grocery Store Seafood

Center for Food Safety. (2025). Mercury bigger worry than radiation in tuna.
Condor Ferries. (2024). Marine & ocean pollution statistics &

facts 2025.
EPA. (2025). Fish and shellfish program newsletter: June 2025.
FDA. (2025). FDA increases scrutiny of imported seafood, papaya, candy and more.
Food Safety News. (2025). Data gaps identified as part of toxins in seafood work.
Food-Safety.com. (2025). 10-year analysis of fish Salmonella outbreaks underlines need for more surveillance.
Global Seafood Alliance. (2025). Responsible seafood summit insights.
IMARC Group. (2024). Fish farming market size, share | forecast report 2033.
National Park Service. (2022). How does mercury reach pristine lakes?
NIH. (2019). Review on natural preservatives for extending fish shelf life.
NOAA Fisheries. (2023). Feeds for aquaculture.
ScienceDirect. (2025). Contaminants in fish and seafood from the marine environment.
Statista. (2025). Fish & seafood—Worldwide | Statista market forecast.
Veterinary Digital. (2024). Preservatives for fish destined for the production of fishmeal.
WHO. (2025). Estimating the burden of foodborne diseases.
Yale Medicine. (2025). Are ultraprocessed foods bad for your health?

Chapter 7: Waxed, Washed, and Worse: Grocery Fruit Exposed

"Additives in processed foods as a potential source of endocrine disruption." PMC, 2024.

"America's vanishing nutrients: Decline in fruit and vegetable nutrition." Rockdustlocal.com, 2024.□

"An alarming decline in the nutritional quality of foods." PMC, 2024.

"Bisphenol A concentration in canned fruits and vegetables." Nature, 2024.

"Declining fruit and vegetable nutrient composition." ASHS Journals, 2009.

"Food additives in fruit processing." Wiley, 2006.

"Foods that contain banned Red Dye 3." HuffPost, 2025.

"Fruits and vegetables aren't as nutritious as they used to be." Yahoo, 2025.□

"Is it safe to eat the sticker on fruit?" SimplyRecipes, 2023.

"Maraschino cherries: 6 downsides to eating them." Healthline, 2019.

"Organophosphorus pesticide contaminants in fruits and vegetables." ScienceDirect, 2023.

"Pesticide residues in fresh fruit and vegetables from farm to fork." PMC, 2022.

"Produce-associated foodborne disease outbreaks, USA, 1998–2013." PMC, 2018.

"Why modern food lost its nutrients." BBC, 2018.

Chapter 8: Tainted Greens and Fruits: The Grocery's Hidden Dangers

"A ten-year survey of bacterial pathogens in fresh, unprocessed food." ScienceDirect, 2025.

"Assessment of bacterial and parasitic contamination of fruits." Frontiers, 2024.

"Bibliographies: 'Irradiation of food.'" Grafiati, 2022.□

"Field study of parasitic contamination of fruits, vegetables and leafy greens." F1000Research, 2024.

"Food contaminants in fruits and vegetables." Taylor & Francis, 2024.

"Food irradiation: An effective but under-utilized technique for food preservation." NIH, 2022.

"Food irradiation research and technology." Wiley Online Books, 2012.

"Growth of human pathogens within fruits and vegetables." FDA, 2022.

"Heavy metals in foods and beverages: Global situation, health implications, and monitoring." PMC, 2023.

"Heavy metals in the vegetables collected from production sites." PMC, 2013.

"Investigation of heavy metal accumulation in vegetables and health risk assessment." Frontiers, 2022.

"Microbial contamination of fruit and vegetables and the behaviour of foodborne pathogens." Academic Oxford, 2008.

"Microbial contamination, an increasing threat to the consumption of fresh fruits and vegetables." Wiley, 2020.

"Parasitic contamination of fruits and vegetables collected from selected local markets of Addis Ababa, Ethiopia." PMC, 2020.
"Pesticide residue monitoring and food safety bibliography." Cornell eCommons, 2024.
"Pesticide residues in food." World Health Organization, 2025.
"Produce safety best practices guide for retailers." FMI, 2025.
"Public health implications of pesticide residues in food: Risks and management." journals, 2024.

Chapter 9: The Milky Mirage: Poisons in Your Carton

"Analysis: Dairy products led global food recalls in first quarter of..." Food-Safety.com, 2025.
"Assessing microplastic contamination in milk and dairy products." Nature, 2025.
"Assessment of milk contamination, associated risk factors, and drug sensitivity patterns among isolated bacteria from raw milk." Wiley, 2022.
"Consumer concerns about hormones in food." Cornell eCommons, 2022.
"Contaminants in the cow's milk we consume? Pasteurization and..." PMC, 2022.□
"Exploring the types of additives in dairy products: A review." IARConsortium, 2024.
"Heavy metal and pesticide levels in dairy products." PubMed, 2020.
"Heavy metals and trace elements in milk and dairy products." Taylor & Francis, 2025.

"Microbial contamination in milk quality and health risk of the consumers of raw milk and dairy products." Semanticscholar, 2019.
"Microplastics and endocrine-disrupting byproducts in infant formula." ScienceDirect, 2025.
"Microplastics in dairy products and human breast milk." ScienceDirect, 2025.
"Nano- and microplastics migration from plastic food packaging into dairy products." PMC, 2023.
"Preservatives | Handbook of dairy foods analysis." Taylor & Francis, 2024.
"Production-related contaminants (Pesticides, antibiotics and. .." NIH, 2019.
"Simultaneous determination of preservatives in dairy products by chromatography." PMC, 2017.

Chapter 10: Sick by the Slice: The Bread That Breaks Our Bodies

"Adverse reactions to wheat or wheat components." PubMed, 2019.
"Assessment of health risks from potassium bromate and trace metals in industrial bread." ScienceDirect, 2022.
"Beneath the crust: The chemical cocktail in our daily bread." Sourdough.co.uk, 2024.
"Chemical contamination in bread from food processing and its health risk assessment." PMC, 2022.
"Evaluation of shelf life and technological properties of bread

supplemented with lactic acid bacteria." ScienceDirect, 2023.
"Glyphosate, pathways to modern diseases II: Celiac sprue and gluten intolerance." PMC, 2013.
"Human health risk assessment of arsenic and potentially toxic elements in bread." PLOS ONE, 2025.
"Industrial bread composition: Potential implications for patients with inflammatory bowel diseases." PMC, 2025.
"Perspective: Refined grains and health: Genuine risk, or guilt by association?" ScienceDirect, 2019.
"Potassium bromate: 50 years of research shows serious health risks." US Right to Know, 2025.
"Review: Does wheat make us fat and sick?" ScienceDirect.com.
"Rustgi, S., Shewry, P. R., & Brouns, F. (2020). Health hazards associated with wheat and gluten consumption in susceptible individuals and status of research on dietary therapies." In Igrejas, G., Ikeda, T. M., & Guzmán, C. (Eds.), *Wheat Quality for Improving Processing and Human Health* (pp. 471-515). Springer. **https://doi.org/10.1007/978-3-030-34163-3_20**
"Separating the empirical wheat from the pseudoscientific chaff." PMC, 2020.
"The two faces of wheat." Frontiers in Nutrition, 2020.
"Wheat flour constituents: How they impact bread quality, and how to modify their functionality." ScienceDirect, 2022.
"Wheat intolerance might be due to glyphosate—new study." Detoxproject.org, 2023.

Why modern wheat is making us sick. Chelsea Green Publishing, 2025.

Chapter 11: Sweeteners and Sugar

"Artificial sweetener annotated bibliography." sdcoi.org.
"Aspartame: A sweet illusion backed by industry pressure." Foodwatch, 2025.
"Aspartame: When lobbying dictates science." Yuka, 2025.
"A brief history of aspartame." Perfy, 2025.
"The curious case of aspartame: How the same evidence can yield opposite conclusions." Food and Drug Law Institute, 2024.
"Effects of artificial and natural sweeteners on host metabolic health." ScienceDirect, 2025.
"Food sweeteners: Angels or clowns for human health?" ScienceDirect, 2024.
"Five sneaky sources of sugar." National Kidney Foundation, 2025.
"Health effects of the use of non-sugar sweeteners: A systematic review." WHO, 2022.
"Hidden sugar and its bitter obstacles." DigitalCommons@URI, 2020.
"Impact of different adulterants on honey quality." ScienceDirect, 2024.
"Low-calorie sweeteners." The Nutrition Source, Harvard, 2025.
"Artificial sweeteners and risk of cardiovascular diseases." BMJ,

2022.
"Artificial sweeteners: A systematic review of metabolic effects in youth." PMC, 2003.
"Artificial sweeteners: History and new concepts on inflammation." PMC, 2021.
"Artificial sweeteners: Sugar-free, but at what cost?" Harvard Health, 2020.
"Artificial sweeteners: A systematic review of metabolic effects in youth." PMC, 2003.
"Spotting hidden sugars in everyday foods." CDC, 2024.
"Sugar substitutes." Research Starters, EBSCO, 2014.
"The toxic impact of honey adulteration: A review." PMC, 2020.

Chapter 12: Bakery and Ready-to-Eat Foods

"Azo dyes and human health: A review." PubMed, 2016.
"Bakery product foodborne illness outbreaks." Foodborne Outbreak Online Database, Marler Clark, 2025.
"Clean label in bread." PMC, 2021.
"Distribution and co-occurrence of food additives in pre-packaged foods." ScienceDirect, 2024.
"E 310 propyl gallate." Ataman Kimya, 2009.
"Effects of freezing rate on frozen bakery dough." ScienceDirect, 2016.
"Evaluation of microbial contamination and chemical qualities of cream-filled pastries." NIH, 2016.
"FDA: Imported pastries linked to Salmonella outbreak."

CIDRAP, 2025.
"Food additives and health." The Nutrition Source, Harvard, 2025.
"Food additives in cakes, biscuits may increase type 2 diabetes risk." Medical News Today, 2024.
"Food additives in fruit processing." Wiley, 2006.
"Functional additives for bakery foods." Clyde E. Stauffer, Springer, 1990.
"Pastries blamed for 100 staph cases." CIDRAP, 2010.
"Propyl gallate." NIH, 2014.
"Propylene glycol in baked goods?" BakerPedia, 2024.
"The health impact of food additives." ERC, 2022.
"Where is Red 40 banned?" Imbarex, 2025.

Chapter 13: Cooking Oils and Fats

"Artificial trans fats banned in U.S." Harvard School of Public Health, 2024.
"Exposure to cooking oil fumes and oxidative damages." PMC, 2012.
"Formation pathways of aldehydes from heated cooking oils." RSC, 2023.
"Hard to digest foods: Are you ready for some surprises?" Julie Nutrition, 2025.
"Health effects of various edible vegetable oils: An umbrella review." ScienceDirect, 2024.
"Hexane extraction of vegetable oils." Anderson International, 2023.

"Industrial vegetable oils show dangerous levels of toxic elements." News-Medical, 2024.
"Influence of omega n-6/n-3 ratio on cardiovascular disease." ScienceDirect, 2024.
"Omega n-6/n-3 ratio on cardiovascular disease." ScienceDirect, 2024.
"Seeding doubt: The truth about cooking oils." Harvard Health, 2025.
"Seed oil extraction using hexane." Maratek, 2024.
"Seed oils: Are they actually toxic?" Cleveland Clinic Health, 2025.
"Seed oils and your health." Stanford Medicine, 2025.
"Seed oils' health effects." Johns Hopkins Public Health, 2025.□
"The 5 most toxic substances in the oilfield industry." Lapeze & Johns, 2018.
"Understanding hexane extraction of vegetable oils." Anderson International, 2023.

Chapter 14: Coffee, Tea, and Beverages

"Bisphenol A leaching from polycarbonate baby bottles into baby food." E-CEP, 2022.
"Bisphenol A migration and associated health risk in polyethylene bottles." Nature, 2025.
"Bisphenol A release from food and beverage containers—A review." PMC, 2023.
"BPA in food." EDF, 2024.
"Chemical insight into pros and cons of coffees from different

regions." Nature, 2025.
"Current status and health risk assessment of heavy metals in tea and tea plantation soils." NIH, 2023.
"Dark side of energy drinks: A comprehensive review." PMC, 2023.
"Energy drink consumption: Beneficial and adverse health effects." PMC, 2005.
"Exposure to endocrine disrupting chemicals from beverage packaging." ScienceDirect, 2024.
"Facile analysis of mycotoxin in coffee and tea samples using a novel IS-FaMEx method." PMC, 2023.
"First evidence of microplastics and their characterization in bottled water." Frontiers, 2023.
"Health effects and public health concerns of energy drink consumption." Frontiers, 2017.
"Health risk assessment of heavy metals in black tea infusion by consumption in adult population." Wiley, 2024.
"Heavy metals in tea." Nature, 2025.
"Main microbiological pollutants of bottled waters and beverages." PMC, 2019.
"Mycotoxin analysis in coffee and tea." PMC, 2023.
"Occurrence, exposure and health risk assessment of heavy metals in tea." Nature, 2025.
"Phthalates and heavy metals as endocrine disruptors in food." ScienceDirect, 2025.
"Quantitative assessment of heavy metal contamination in instant coffee." PAOM, 2022.

"Rethink bottled water's huge and growing toll on human health." BMJ Group, 2024.□
"Tea leaves can steep away lead, study finds." NY Times, 2025.
"The benefits and risks of consuming brewed tea: Beware of toxic elements and contaminants." PMC, 2013.
"Urgent rethink of bottled water's huge and growing toll on human health." BMJ Group, 2024.□
"A worldwide systematic review of ochratoxin A in various coffee." Taylor & Francis, 2024.

Chapter 15: Spices, Condiments, and Hidden Ingredients

"48 food additives to avoid—Could these be in your diet?" IAWP Wellness Coach, 2022.
"Additives in processed foods." Ohio State Health & Discovery, 2022.
"Artificial food additives: Hazardous to long-term health?" PubMed, 2024.
"The effects of condiments on your health." WebMD, 2024.
"Food additives and health." The Nutrition Source, Harvard, 2025.
"Herbs and spices as functional food ingredients." ScienceDirect, 2025.
"History of spices." McCormick Science Institute, 2025.
"A comprehensive review of spices: Use of prevalent preservative techniques and bio-preservatives for enhancing shelf life of spices." Nutrition and Food Processing, 2024.
"Spices as sustainable food preservatives: A comprehensive re-

view of their antimicrobial potential." PMC, 2023.
"Toxicological effect of monosodium glutamate in seasonings on health." IRIS Publishers, 2019.
"What's in your food? 100+ food additives explained." ZOE, 2025.□
"What's really in your spice jar? A deep dive into additives, fillers." Salice Seasoning, 2025.□
"Your herbs and spices might contain arsenic, cadmium & lead." Consumer Reports, 2023.

Chapter 16: Supplements and "Health" Foods

"Combating deception in dietary supplement advertising." FTC, 2013.
"Dangerous dietary supplements and false advertising claims." Ryan Law Group, 2024.
"Daily ingestion of protein bars (with or without added fiber) impacts microbiota and gut function." ScienceDirect, 2025.
"Hundreds of supplements have undeclared, potentially harmful ingredients." US Pharmacist, 2018.
"Is your diet natural? 7 hidden chemicals in 'healthy' foods." NaturesTrunk, 2025.□
"The hidden dangers of dietary supplements." Harvard Health, 2025.
"The hidden dangers of protein powders." Harvard Health, 2022.
"The hidden problems with protein bars—And what to have instead." Kaged, 2024.

"Purity Products announces recall on the dietary supplement." FDA, 2025.
"Protein powders may be doing more harm than good." Center for Research, 2025.
"Protein powders and shakes contain high levels of lead." Consumer Reports, 2025.
"Protein bars might not give you the health boost you think." Health, 2025.
"Recalls of foods & dietary supplements." FDA, 2024.
"Supplement recalled by FDA classified as 'deadly'." Prevention, 2025.□
"The truth about vitamins and supplements: Are they helpful or harmful?" Baylor Scott & White Health, 2025.
"Unapproved pharmaceutical ingredients included in dietary supplements." NIH, 2018.
"Undeclared ingredients in supplements." US Pharmacist, 2018.
"Why scientists found lead in protein powders." C&EN, 2025.

Chapter 17: Baby Food, Infant Formula, Snacks, and Sippy-Cup Surprises

"AAP: Babies should eat a varied diet to protect against heavy metals." AAP, 2022.
"ADHD and heavy metals: ADHD baby food lawsuit." Wisner Baum, 2025.
"Baby food labels will reveal levels of lead and other heavy metals." CNN, 2025.

"Baby foods: Smooth, sweet, and poorly aligned with health recommendations." News-Medical.net, 2025.

"Concentrations of heavy metals in processed baby foods and infant formula: A worldwide scoping review." Academic.oup.com, 2025.

"Healthy baby food—What's in my baby's food?" HBBF, 2022.□

"Heavy metals in baby food: Reducing risk of exposure." HealthyChildren.org/Academy of Pediatrics, 2025.

"I'm a microplastics researcher. Here's how to limit their dangers." UCSF.edu, 2024.□

"Infant formula recall prompted by 13 cases of infant botulism." AAP, 2025.

"Infant formula: Safety do's and don'ts." FDA, 2023.□

"Investigation of Cronobacter infections from powdered infant formula." FDA, 2022.

"Microplastic release from the degradation of polypropylene feeding bottles." Nature, 2020.

"Microplastics and endocrine-disrupting byproducts in infant formula." ScienceDirect, 2025.

"Most baby foods are sweet, smooth, and poorly aligned with health recommendations." News-Medical.net, 2025.

"Outbreak investigation of infant botulism: Infant formula." FDA, 2025.

"Preliminary tests find germ that causes botulism in ByHeart product." ABC, 2025.

"The plastic chemicals hiding in your food." Consumer Re-

ports, 2024.
"Toxic baby food lawsuit | Autism, ADHD & metals (2025)." Sokolove Law, 2025.
"A narrative review of toxic heavy metal content of infant and toddler foods." PMC, 2022.

Chapter 18: Pet Food and Household Items

"Common cleaning products that can harm your pets." PetMD, 2024.
"Contamination of synthetic minerals with heavy metals in pet and livestock feeds." Solutions Pet Products, 2025.
"Evaluation of microbial contamination and chemical qualities of commercial pet foods." NIH, 2016.
"FDA data reveals that 63% of pet food recalls are preventable." Nextbeam, 2025.
"Individual and combined contamination of the toxic metals in imported dog and cat food." PMC, 2025.
"Migration of phthalates and bisphenol A from polyethylene packaging into food." PMC, 2025.
"Pesticide residues in pet food threaten health of companion animals." Beyond Pesticides, 2025.
"Pet food recalls: More than 40% due to Salmonella." Pet Food Industry, 2024.
"Pet food safety at risk? Investigating toxic metal contamination in pet food." RSC, 2025.
"Poisonous household products." ASPCA, 2024.
"Quantification of metals in commercially available cat and dog

food products." ScienceDirect, 2024.
"Toxic element levels in ingredients and commercial pet foods." Nature, 2021.
"Toxic pet food contaminants: Arsenic, BPA, PCB, aflatoxin." Pet Food Industry, 2022.
"Evaluation of arsenic, cadmium, lead, and mercury contamination in commercial dog foods." PMC, 2018.
"Determination of bisphenol A in commercial cat food marketed in the Czech Republic." PMC, 2021.

Chapter 19: Water and Ice

"Bottled water brands to avoid." Concord Longevity Medicine, 2025.
"Bottled water drinkers ingest more microplastics." Fox News, 2025.
"Bottled water in America mostly tap." NY Rural Water, 2023.
"Expired water safety." Business Insider, 2023.
"FDA vs EPA—Bottled water." IBWA, 2025.
"First evidence of microplastics and their characterization in bottled water." Frontiers, 2023.
"Forever chemicals in US water." EESI, 2024.
"Long-term risks: Bottled water." SciTech Daily, 2025.
"Main microbiological pollutants of bottled waters and beverages." PMC, 2019.
"Microplastics in our waters: Concern." Penn State Extension, 2025.
"Occurrence of microplastics in tap/bottled water." PMC,

2022.
"PFAS contamination health risks." EPA, 2025.
"PFAS 'forever chemicals' found in bottled and tap water." Birmingham University, 2024.□
"Research into bottled water contaminants." ScienceDaily, 2025.
"Shelf life of waters." Olympian Water Testing, 2025.
"Tap water PFAS across the US." USGS, 2023.
"Urgent rethink of bottled water's huge and growing toll on human health." BMJ Group, 2024.

Chapter 20: Organic Truths and Grocery Store Myths

"Are you being fooled by 'organic' labels?" Miller IP, 2024.□
"Decoding organic vs. non-organic labels." Banner Peak Health, 2025.
"Difference between organic & natural labels in USA." TangieCo, 2025.
"Food fraud explosion: Tenfold increase 2020–2024." DIGICOMPLY, 2024.
"Fraudulent organic certificates." USDA, 2023.
"Gap between select organic and conventional produce prices." USDA ERS, 2025.
"Ingredients allowed in non-organic portion of organic foods." USDA, 2023.
"Labeling organic products." USDA Agricultural Marketing Service, 2004.
"Natural vs. organic: Does the label matter?" Rodale Institute,

2025.
"Non-organic ingredients allowed under organic label." Beyond Pesticides, 2007.
"Non-organic ingredients in organic foods." HealthCastle.com, 2021.
"Organic 101: What the USDA organic label means." USDA, 2012.
"Organic food fraud: Some surprises." Real Organic Project, 2021.
"Organic foods: Are they safer? More nutritious?" Mayo Clinic, 2025.
"Organic vs. conventional food prices." LendingTree, 2025.
"USDA amends the national list of allowed and prohibited substances." MNCIA, 2022.
"USDA allows 38 non-organic ingredients in foods labeled organic." Beyond Pesticides, 2007.
"What ingredients can be utilized in the 5% of non-organic allowed in organic food?" USDA, 2023.

Chapter 21: The Great Farmers Market Deception

California Department of Food and Agriculture. (2014). Farmers Market Inspection Program: 2014 Annual Report.
Farmers Market Coalition. (2014). Fraud in the Market: An Examination of Vendor Misrepresentation at Farmers Markets. Scholarship Repository, Florida State University Law School.
Iowa District Court, Northern District. (2017). United States

v. Randy Constant, Case No. 17-cr-03043.
Los Angeles County Department of Public Health. (2013). Farmers Market Vendor Violations: Annual Enforcement Summary.
Pennsylvania Department of Agriculture. (2013). Farmers Market Nutrition Program Voucher Analysis: Reseller Capture Rates.
U.S. House of Representatives Committee on Oversight and Government Reform. (2010). Seafood Marketing: Combating Fraud and Deception. Congressional Research Service Report RL34124.
Virginia Department of Agriculture and Consumer Services. (2012). Farmers Market Reselling Study: Patterns of Wholesale Produce Acquisition.

Government and Academic Sources

California Department of Food and Agriculture. (2014). *Farmers Market Inspection Program: 2014 Annual Report*. (Documenting $1 million allocation for fraud investigations under Assembly Bill 1871).
Farmers Market Coalition. (2014). *Fraud in the Market: An Examination of Vendor Misrepresentation at Farmers Markets*. Scholarship Repository, Florida State University Law School.
Iowa District Court, Northern District. (2017). *United States v. Randy Constant*, Case No. 17-cr-03043. (Documenting 11 million bushels of fraudulently marketed organic grain, 2010-2017).

Los Angeles County Department of Public Health. (2013). *Farmers Market Vendor Violations: Annual Enforcement Summary*. (Citing 19 vendors fined for misrepresentation).

Pennsylvania Department of Agriculture. (2013). *Farmers Market Nutrition Program Voucher Analysis: Reseller Capture Rates*. (Finding resellers captured 90% of voucher value).

U.S. House of Representatives Committee on Oversight and Government Reform. (2010). *Seafood Marketing: Combating Fraud and Deception*. Congressional Research Service Report RL34124.

Virginia Department of Agriculture and Consumer Services. (2012). *Farmers Market Reselling Study: Patterns of Wholesale Produce Acquisition*.

Chapter 22 and others

American Community Gardening Association. (Various years). Community Gardening Resources. Retrieved from **https://communitygarden.org**

U.S. Department of Agriculture. (2024). Urban Agriculture Toolkit. Retrieved from **https://usda.gov**

Harvard T.H. Chan School of Public Health. (2024). Fermented Foods and Health. Retrieved from **https://hsph.harvard.edu**

Yale Medicine. (2025). Are Ultra-Processed Foods Bad for Your Health? Retrieved from **https://yalemedicine.org**

Stanford Medicine. (2025). Ultra-Processed Food: Five Things to Know. Retrieved from **https://med.stanford.edu**

Cooperative Grocer Network. (2023). How Food Co-ops Work. Retrieved from **https://grocer.coop**

National Sustainable Agriculture Coalition. (2024). Guide to Community Supported Agriculture. Retrieved from **https://sustainableagriculture.net**

U.S. Environmental Protection Agency. (2024). Reducing Plastic Use in the Home. Retrieved from **https://epa.gov**American Community Gardening Association. Various years. Community Gardening Resources.

USDA. 2024. Urban Agriculture Toolkit.

Harvard T.H. Chan School of Public Health. 2024. Fermented Foods and Health.

Yale Medicine. 2025. Are Ultra-Processed Foods Bad for Your Health?

Stanford Medicine. 2025. Ultra-Processed Food: Five Things to Know.

Cooperative Grocer Network. 2023. How Food Co-ops Work.

National Sustainable Agriculture Coalition. 2024. Guide to Community Supported Agriculture.

EPA. 2024. Reducing Plastic Use in the Home.

Investigative Journalism and News Reports

CBC Marketplace. (2017). *Farmers Market Lies Exposed: Hidden Camera Investigation*. Canadian Broadcasting Corporation.

Forbes. (2021). *Simple Lessons About Ad Fraud From the Farmers' Market.* (May 31, 2021).
Mashed. (2018). *Your Favorite Farmers Market Might Be a Scam.* (August 22, 2018).
NBC4 Los Angeles. (2014). *Farmers Market Fraud: Undercover Investigation.* KNBC-TV Investigative Reports.
Perishable Pundit. (2011). *Fraudulent Farmer's Markets Detrimental to Legitimate Farms, Retailers and Consumers.* (February 8, 2011).
The Daily Dot. (2024). *Are Farmer's Market Vendors Scamming You? Here's How to Tell.* (July 5, 2024).
Voice of San Diego. (2013). *When Fraud Hits the Farmers Market.* (April 8, 2013).
Vox. (2016). *Think You're Eating Local Food? It Might Be a Lie.* (April 13, 2016).

Consumer Advocacy and Industry Sources

Ecology Center. (2024). *A Matter of Trust and Vigilance: Re-Selling at Farmers Markets.* (July 2, 2024).
Farm Forward. (2024). *Dairy Deception: Corruption and Consumer Fraud.* (April 28, 2024).
Foodwise. (2022). *California Takes a Bite Out of Farmers Market Fraud.* (November 4, 2022).
Non-GMO Report. (2023). *Fraud is "Unquestionably, the Biggest Threat to Organic".* (September 6, 2023).
OrganicEye. (2025). *USDA Organic Certification "Untrustworthy".* (May 18, 2025).

Organic Farmers Association. (2020). *The Tragedy of Fraud.* (August 12, 2020).

Real Organic Project. (2023). *Peter Whoriskey Uncovering Fraud in Organic Meat, Milk, Eggs and Grain.* Podcast Episode Six.

Reddit r/Costco. (2022). *Am I Crazy or Is a Local Baker Selling Costco Cookies at the Farmers Market?* (July 16, 2022).

Reddit r/Scams. (2024). *Farmers Market Scam Makes Me Mad.* (September 3, 2024).

YouTube: Consumer Beware. (2020). *FARMERS MARKET EXPOSED | Food Fraud.* (February 3, 2020).

YouTube: Farmer Exposé. (2025). *99% of Your 'Healthy' Eggs & Meat Are a Scam!* (June 22, 2025).

YouTube: Hidden Camera Investigation. (2017). *Farmers Market Lies Exposed.* (September 28, 2017).

Chapter Twenty-Six

Further Reading

MAIN COLLECTION: BOOKS BY Marko Vovk

Poisoned at the Grocery Store: Why Shopping Fresh Is Not Enough to Escape a Toxic Food Supply

Surviving Electrosmog: How to Understand and Reduce Invisible Pollution in Your Home and Life

Forever Chemicals: How PFAS Pollutes Our Blood and Lives

Avoid Waterproofing, Drain Cleaning and Foundation Repair Scams

Childless Cat Lady: Movement, Dynamics, Health, and Political Influence

Deep Down the Rabbit Hole Poetry

Don't Rent This Home, Condo, or Apartment

Empty Cradles: Declining Birth Rates Explained

Fix Your Toxic Home and Live Longer

Make Your Home Great Again (For Homeowners and Buyers) & Expanded Tips Edition

Nuclear Extinction Event Is Killing Our Families

Pets: The Hidden Costs of Companionship

Poisoned at the Grocery Store

Project 2025 Quick Review

The Sixth Extinction: Return to Earth 2225
The Water You Drink May Be Killing You
No-Mow Living: The Real Hidden Costs of Grass
BIAS: How Our Minds Deceive Us – 18 Ways Your Perceptions Are Skewed and How to See More Clearly

Earth Helpers Kids' Series
PFAS KIDS: The Forever Chemical Mystery
The Great Smoke, Fire & Dust Adventure
EMF KIDS: The Secret World of Invisible Waves
Nuclear KIDS: Little Lessons from Atomic Power
Grass KIDS: Why the Lawn Isn't Always Greener
Home Safety KIDS: Smart Habits for Everyday Dangers
Lucky To Be Alive: Discover Why Every Life Is a Miracle
The Vitamin ABC's: A Healthy Kids Guide

Eight additional Earth Helper Series titles coming 2026–2027.
Find all titles online by searching "Marko Vovk" on Amazon.

Made in the USA
Monee, IL
04 November 2026

67381909R00134